POCKET GUIDE TO
Home Health
Care

DATE DUE

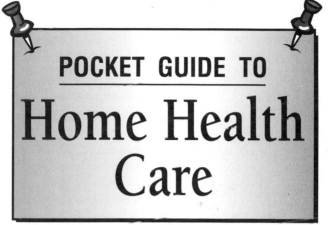

POCKET GUIDE TO
Home Health Care

Karen McGough Monks, MSN, RN

Recruitment Staff Development Specialist
Yuma Regional Home Care
Yuma, Arizona

W.B. SAUNDERS COMPANY
A Harcourt Health Sciences Company
Philadelphia   London   Toronto   Montreal   Sydney   Tokyo

DEC 1 8 2001

W.B. SAUNDERS COMPANY
A Harcourt Health Sciences Company

The Curtis Center
Independence Square West
Philadelphia, Pennsylvania 19106

Library of Congress Cataloging-in-Publication Data

Monks, Karen McGough
  Pocket guide to home health care / Karen McGough Monks

  p. cm.

  Includes bibliographical references

  ISBN 0–7216–8558–7

  1. Home care services—Handbooks, manuals, etc.
  [DNLM: 1. Home Care Services—Handbooks. WY
  49 M745p 2000]

  RA645.35 .M66 2000   362.1′4—dc21

                                          99–044468

POCKET GUIDE TO HOME
HEALTH CARE   ISBN 0–7216–8558–7

Printed in the United States of America

Last digit is the print number: 9 8 7 6 5 4 3 2 1

To my husband, Patrick,
for all of your support and encouragement

Reviewers

Judith Bailey, BSN, MBA
San Diego State University and National University
San Diego, California

Rick Douden, RPTA
Anderson Area Medical Center
Anderson, South Carolina

Deborah Evers, MSN, RN
Mercy Hospital of Pittsburgh and South Hills Health
  System Home Health Agency
Pittsburgh, Pennsylvania

Christine Frontera, OTR/L
AnMed Home Health Agency
Anderson, South Carolina

Roxanne O'Hearn, RPT, BS
St. Luke's Hospital
Duluth, Minnesota

Tamala Dykes Paxton, RN,C, MS
Delaware Technical Community College
Georgetown, Delaware

Jeanie Stoker, BSN, RN,C, MPA
AnMed Health Systems and AnMed Home
  Care Services
Anderson, South Carolina

Preface

Nurses and therapists move into the home health care field for the first time every year. Some receive comprehensive orientation to their new positions, but others receive limited orientation. Even with comprehensive orientation, the practitioners new to home health care could still benefit from a reference that reinforces the content addressed during orientation. Some excellent references are published for the home health care practitioner, but they do not contain the detailed guidance and basic information needed to meet state and federal requirements. This book, *Pocket Guide to Home Health Care,* is designed to meet these needs. It is not intended to take the place of a comprehensive orientation but to supplement that orientation.

Pocket Guide to Home Health Care is also designed to provide a user-friendly reference for home health care professionals that can be used at their homes and can be carried in the car so it is available during visits. The content and design are based upon feedback from experienced home health care professionals. Many have stated that they wish they had a similar reference when they began their careers in home health care.

Practitioners new to home health care are not the only ones who will benefit from this pocket guide. Experienced home health care practitioners, students in nursing, physical therapy, occupational therapy, and speech pathology, and case managers for third-party payors, hospitals, and skilled nursing facilities will also find the information useful.

It does not take long for the new home health care professional to become acutely aware of the practice differences between home health care and acute or extended health care. This pocket guide begins by discussing those differences. Unlike acute and extended health care, the home health care practitioner is responsible for assessing clients for ongoing eligibility to receive home health care and for documenting that eligibility. Chapter 3 presents the Medicare Conditions of Participation (COP) for home health care agencies that is the basis for home health care practice. This discussion includes the home health care practitioner's responsibilities in relation to regulations. *Pocket Guide to Home Health Care* also includes information about changes in the home health care professional's responsibilities in regard to data gathering for the Outcome and Assessment Information Set (OASIS).

Examples for implementation and documentation of the Conditions of Participation, which is crucial for maintaining compliance with Medicare regulations, are offered throughout the book. Basic information about safety, infection control, ethical issues, and legal aspects as they relate to home health care is also included.

Since home health care regulations are in continuous flux, extra margin space is provided in the conditions of participation and documentation chapters to add updated information. Tables that highlight crucial and frequently used information are provided throughout the pocket guide for ready reference. Field Tips, a special feature, emphasize important information to provide additional guidance for the novice home health care practitioner.

KAREN MCGOUGH MONKS

Acknowledgment

In appreciation to Gail Schilling, BSN, RN,C, for sharing her home health care expertise.

Contents

APPENDIX B

Home Health Care Professional

1

This chapter provides an overview of home health care, including the role of the home health professional and the differences in practice of the professional in the home versus in acute and long-term care facilities.

PURPOSE OF BOOK

The purpose of this book is to provide a handbook to be used as a ready reference for the nurse or therapist who is making the transition from work in an acute or long-term care facility to home care. It is not intended to be a substitute for a comprehensive orientation program to home health care but as a supplement to that program. This book also is useful for the experienced home health case manager and for nursing students who are participating in a home health experience in their nursing programs. The book is designed so that nurses and therapists can carry it with them in the car to be used as a handy resource while making home visits.

Home care practice is a much different experience for the professional than that found in either acute or long-term care facilities. Because of the different nature of home care practice, newly oriented professionals may have unsuccessfully searched for resources to provide guidance in their practice. Until recently, most basic nursing and therapy programs have not devoted much time to home health care in their curricula. It usually takes 6 to 12 months to adapt to the role of a case manager in home health care. This is an area in which practitioners new to home care have had little experience. The materials in this book have proven to be a beneficial resource for new home health practitioners during orientation to a home health agency. These materials have been refined based on feedback from home health nurses and therapists who are currently working in the field.

Most other books written for the home health professional contain valuable information; however, many references assume that the individual already has a working knowledge of the basic information needed to function in the field. The expectations of the home health staff are very different from those in other types of health care facilities. Professionals who work in acute care and extended care facilities have administrators and managers readily available to make sure that the patients meet Medicare eligibility criteria and that other regulations are observed. In home health, nurses and therapists are responsible for assessing and documenting the clients' conditions to determine their eligibility for home care and to track their continuing eligibility.

A home health agency depends on the home care professional's record keeping to justify reimbursement for services and to document that the agency remains in compliance with all of the regulations that govern home health. Hospitals and skilled nursing facilities do not have to submit related documentation when billing for reimbursement; whereas, home health agencies are frequently required to submit field staff visit notes.

Chapter 2 explains the various types of managed care and payor sources for home care. Chapter 3 discusses Medicare's Conditions of Participation (COP) that are required of home health agencies to maintain their Medicare certification so they can receive reimbursement for the services they provide. These are the requirements that the home health professionals are responsible for when assisting their agencies to remain in compliance with Medicare COPs. Most third-party payors other than Medicare use the COPs as guidelines to determine their own requirements for reimbursement of services.

This chapter lays the basis for the remainder of the book. The rest of the book discusses ways to implement the COPs and other regulatory requirements. Practical examples are given for these various implementations. The book also discusses other aspects of health care such as infection control and legal and ethical issues and how they vary in the practice of home care.

COMPARISONS BETWEEN HOME CARE AND ACUTE EXTENDED CARE

The home care professional needs to possess the same basic skills as does the nurse or therapist who works in acute and extended care facilities. There are additional skills, that are quite different, that the home health professional is expected to exercise. In home health care, practitioners are expected to function more independently than they do in acute or extended care facilities. This chapter discusses how those skills are adapted for home health care.

Two major skills that are crucial in caring for patients in their homes as well as in structured facilities are assessment and teaching. No matter what the client's primary diagnosis, both of these skills are always necessary. The major difference is that in home care you are performing these skills in the client's home and do not always have supplies readily available to perform them. The successful home health professional learns to improvise based on what materials are available.

Another difference is that there is usually only one or two professionals working with a given client and family. You cannot depend on someone else picking up on a part of the assessment or instruction that you may have missed. On the other hand, this situation provides more consistency for the client.

Some newly oriented home care professionals experience anxiety at the thought of caring for clients in the home environment. These environments are uncontrolled and sometimes unstable. The client and family, not the health care provider, control the environment. The focus is on families and communities as opposed to just the individual client. The good news is that the majority of clients are most appreciative of the care provided. They marvel that you would take the time to come to their homes to assist them. Field staff members are surprised at how receptive the client and family are to the care that is rendered.

Home care seems to be one of those areas of practice that the practitioner either really loves or really hates. Most nurses and therapists tend to enjoy home health practice once they have adjusted to the different practice environment. The professionals who do not seem to ever adjust to home care seem to be ones who have a hard time practicing without the technology and equipment found in health care facilities.

At first the scope of accountability in home care can be intimidating. Nurses and therapists are not only responsible for the care that is rendered during a visit but also must follow up on events that occur when they are not present. Some practitioners feel uncomfortable when they cannot keep an eye on what is happening to the client on a regular basis. Home health professionals need to develop a strong skill to assess the abilities and needs of the client and the family caregiver and to trust that they will be able to carry through on instructions. Sometimes we do not give the clients and their families sufficient credit for their own abilities and resources.

At first, new practitioners experience anxiety in home health because they are moving from an environment where they feel self-confident. One becomes proficient, competent, and knowledgeable once she/he has adjusted to a certain work environment. It takes a certain amount of courage to move to a new work environment. We always experience anxiety when we take on a new job, but that is how we can grow professionally. After we become adjusted, we will find that we again have that old self-confidence and can enjoy the work.

Most agencies recognize the value of assigning a preceptor to each new employee. If your agency does not have a formal preceptor program, seek out one or two home care professionals in your discipline for guidance. Do not be afraid to ask questions. You will find that most of the staff members will remember what it was like to be new to home health. You will also find that even seasoned staff members are still asking questions. Requirements change frequently enough that everyone is continuously learning. Don't let this statement intimidate you, but on the other hand never think that you know so much that you no longer need to keep up to date.

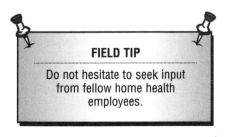

FIELD TIP

Do not hesitate to seek input from fellow home health employees.

It is usually recommended that nurses and therapists have at least one year of experience in a structured facility before they work in home health. This recommendation is because of the independent nature of the practice in home health. The home care professional is not going to have a colleague as readily available as in a structured facility so that a solid basic experience is valuable. That basic experience will help instill the needed self-confidence in your skills.

Work schedules tend to be flexible. The individual practitioner will establish the schedule based on the needs of the clients but can also work around his/her personal and family schedules. The schedules in a structured facility are predetermined. The staff in the hospital work particular shifts, whereas the home health staff may make some visits in the morning and then not need to see a client until later in the day. Some individuals like this flexibility whereas others prefer more structure. This preference should be considered before someone decides to take a home care position.

Assessment Skills

When making assessments, the nurse or therapist needs to assess both the client and the family and home environment. Further, the assessment needs to include the ability and willingness of the client or caregiver to provide the necessary care. The home care practitioner may be the only one seeing the client and family, so assessment and documentation need to be comprehensive. The client assessment in the home tends to focus better on the total client than it does in the acute or extended care setting. This is because the nurse or therapist views the client in his/her own environment and usually has the opportunity to meet other members of the household.

The home health professional has the chance to become familiar with the community where the client lives, its available resources, and the coping skills of both the client and family. A knowledge of the various cultures that exist within the community is required to assess and use community resources effectively.

Teaching Skills

The home health practitioner frequently will be teaching two or more people at a time. When teaching the client and caregiver(s), the practitioner may be the only one teaching that content. The nurse or therapist cannot depend on someone else to reinforce the teaching or pick up any loose ends that might have been missed. On the other hand, the practitioner can have better control over the teaching process and can make sure that all of the needed information is provided. The home care practitioner can provide individualized teaching with relatively few interruptions.

Since clients are being discharged so rapidly from hospitals, teaching that used to take place before discharge is not happening. Home health practitioners have a limited period of time in which to provide instructions, so they need to be efficient with that time. Most people seem to learn better in the environment in which they are going to be using the information. The teaching will be more effective when the nurse or therapist is familiar with the client's home.

The practitioner in an acute or extended care facility does not always know the type of dwelling in which the client lives. For example, the client may not have running water, heat, or air conditioning; therefore, the teaching cannot be adapted to the client's environment. The home care practitioner has the advantage of being right there.

Documentation Skills

Documentation probably poses the greatest challenge to home care professionals. It needs to be precise and reflect not only the client's care and response to the care but also that state, federal, and third-party requirements have been met. The amount of detailed documentation that is needed in home health can be frustrating. The sooner that you learn to be concise in your charting the better you will feel. More agencies are realizing the benefits of using computer programs for documentation to help the field staff become more efficient. Frequently, only one or two practitioners are responsible for all documentation for a given client. There is not another shift to depend on to pick up on areas that you may have missed.

Communication and Collaboration

Home health professional staff members are required to collaborate across all disciplines and organizations more than would be required in other health care areas. Most practitioners enjoy the challenge of home health because each client and family poses different issues to stimulate the nurse's or therapist's creativity. At first, home care practitioners may feel intimidated by the unstructured environment, but they need to remember that there are always resources available to them. Home care practitioners make use of beepers, cellular phones, fax machines, and computers to facilitate communication.

Agencies make sure that there is a supervisor available by telephone. If the question does not need to be answered immediately, the practitioner can stop at the agency later to discuss the problem with his/her supervisor. If a staff member is having a problem with equipment or a procedure such as starting an intravenous (IV) infusion, the agency will arrange for another nurse to come to provide assistance if the problem cannot be solved over the phone. A practitioner is never left completely without assistance. The nurse or therapist should also take advantage of the agency's weekly case conferences where discussion of client situations provides insights into managing client cases effectively.

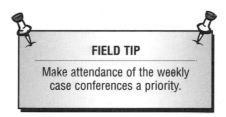

FIELD TIP

Make attendance of the weekly case conferences a priority.

Decision-Making Skills

The decision-making process used when developing the client's plan of care is more of a shared process with the client and family than that which occurs in a structured facility. In a structured facility, the decisions are influenced most by facility protocols and doctors' orders and there is minimal client involvement. In home health, the decision making is shared by the doctor, nurse, therapists, and especially, the client and family.

These decisions are also more influenced by characteristics of the community. Organizations within the community that provide reimbursement for services have varying requirements for eligibility that need to be considered when planning the client's care. There is a better chance for the clients to receive individualized care since they are seen within their own environment. Each client is seen on an individual basis by the agency staff members when there is minimal opportunity for interruptions by other clients and staff.

Case Management Skills

Case management requires proficient communication, negotiation, conflict-resolution, and problem solving skills. Communication is more of a challenge in home care because there is no structured setting in which all the disciplines meet.

Communications with the physician usually take place over the phone. The wise home health professional will make a point of making a doctor's office visit with the client from time to time, especially when the client's care is complicated. Hospital-based nurses and therapists can see the doctor regularly. They come to learn the doctor's expectations in a given situation such as with a dressing change. In the hospital, the doctor is more readily available to clarify orders and answer questions.

Many doctors are just becoming familiar with the advantages of home health care and the regulations that govern it. Home care professionals can help educate physicians about these various regulations. Some ways to involve physicians in home care are to:

    Invite one or two physicians to serve on the agency's professional advisory board
    Ask them for feedback through a questionnaire
    Distribute a brochure to inform them about the agency and the services it provides.

Some physicians indicate that they would appreciate having a limited number of nurses take care of their patients so they are not receiving numerous phone calls from several different nurses from the same agency. This arrangement helps the doctor to get used to a more limited number of nurses and therapists and the staff to become familiar with an individual doctor's practice. Assigning a limited number of professionals to each doctor can be a real challenge, especially if the agency serves a large geographic area. Some physicians are just happy to have phone calls limited from an agency. Depending upon doctor preferences, it may help to use the fax machine for messages or to leave messages so that the doctor can respond to all questions through one supervisor. Of course, this method requires communication with that supervisor so she/he understands what information is needed.

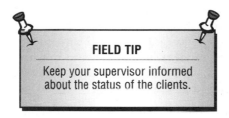

FIELD TIP

Keep your supervisor informed
about the status of the clients.

There are some physicians who will make home health visits that can be reimbursed by Medicare. This practice may increase in the future. To qualify for Medicare reimbursement for the physician's visit, the client must require complex or multidisciplinary care that requires frequent revisions of the plan of care. Some doctors will occasionally make home visits to certain clients without expecting reimbursement.

In the home, clients have a better opportunity to let their wishes be known in relation to their plan of care. Although the logistics of home care complicate communication, it doesn't mean that it is impossible. Each agency schedules case conferences to promote communication within and between the various professionals involved in a client's care. It is up to the individual staff member to take advantage of these case conferences. There are many ways for the staff member to maintain communication with the physician including phone, fax, and office visits.

The home health professional needs to maintain contact with many agencies in the community and even those outside the community that still affect the client's care. In home health, the nurse or therapist is more likely to play the role of client advocate.

This advocacy may take the form of educating clients about available community resources and how to access them; for example, when clients need to purchase a piece of equipment they depend on the agency personnel for information about price ranges. Many times clients will purchase equipment such as a shower bench at a medical supply company for two times the amount for which it can be purchased at a pharmacy.

Clients also require an advocate to communicate with their physicians, other community resources, and any third-party payor case managers that authorize payment for health care services. The home health nurse or therapist, as the individual who sees a client on a frequent basis and is familiar with his/her environment and circumstances, is in the best position to be a client advocate. Many clients do not understand how to work their way through the complex health care system in order to obtain what they need. The home care professional is responsible for providing the needed assistance or for arranging a medical social service referral when the situation is beyond the professional's expertise.

The home health nurse's or therapist's focus will be more on strategies to achieve the client's desired outcomes, whereas the professional in a structured facility focuses on the medical and institutional goals. The length of care for the client in the home is determined by the client's needs, home care professional's assessments, doctor's orders, and third-party payor regulations.

Organization Skills

Another challenge for the home care professional is that resources are not as readily available for client care. The staff member must remember to take all needed supplies with him/her so an unnecessary trip is not made. Organization is crucial for all health care workers, but is even more so for the home health worker. Having to make an extra round trip to the client's home because you forgot to bring an extra syringe or catheter is usually all it takes to remember to be organized. It can be an interesting challenge to learn to adapt your procedures to the home situation and still maintain asepsis. You learn little things such as asking the client to leave the cat outside the bedroom when you are changing a wound dressing.

HOME HEALTH SPECIALTIES

A unique and rewarding aspect of home care is that the professional has the opportunity to provide comprehensive, individualized client care. Home health staff find that providing care in the home is less stressful. There is more opportunity to provide thorough, hands-on care without interruption. You can usually depend on giving the client and family your attention for the time designated for their visit. Clients are being discharged rapidly from acute facilities, so they are coming home sicker and with less time to learn how to care for themselves. The wound care and IV antibiotic therapy that used to be provided in acute care facilities are now being provided in the home. Home health nurses are the ones who have the expertise in wound care rather than the acute care nurses.

The home care nurse or therapist has the opportunity to develop various specialties. Currently, the greatest need is for adult care health professionals, but within that area of practice are opportunities to develop expertise in wound care and IV therapy. Geriatric nursing and therapy are areas of continuing demand in home health. There is a growing appreciation for the benefits of maternal-child visits for the "at risk" new mother and baby. (The at risk mother is usually defined as the unmarried teenage mother.)

Many families of developmentally disabled children are able to care for their children at home if they can receive the benefit of skilled nursing and therapy supervision and respite care. These services are frequently reimbursed by Medicaid or the Department of Economic Security. Enterostomal therapy is another highly used specialty in home care. Psychiatric nursing services can be reimbursed by Medicare as long as those services are provided by a qualified practitioner.

PRACTICE RESOURCES

There are many journals that provide a wealth of information related to home health practice. Additionally, the Internet serves as a resource for up-to-date information without consuming a great deal of time researching at the library. Table 1–1 provides a list of home health journals for nurses and therapists. Table 1–2 provides some Internet sites that could prove beneficial to the home care professional.

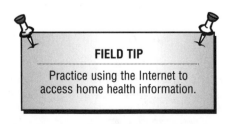

FIELD TIP

Practice using the Internet to access home health information.

Table 1–1	HOME HEALTH CARE JOURNALS

AJOT: The American Journal of Occupational Therapy (American Occupational Therapy Association)

AOTA's OT Week (American Occupational Therapy Association)

Caring Magazine (National Association for Home Care)

Home Care Provider (Mosby, Inc.)

Home Healthcare Nurse: Official Journal of the Home Healthcare Nurses Association (Lippincott)

Home Health Insights (Springhouse Corporation)

Home Health Focus (Mosby, Inc.)

Infection Control Today (Virgo Publications, Inc.)

Issues on Aging: Official Publication of the Section on Geriatrics of the American Physical Therapy Association (APTA)

Journal of Intravenous Nursing: Official Journal of Intravenous Nurses Society (Lippincott-Raven Publishers)

JOSPT: Journal of Orthopedic & Sports Physical Therapy: American Physical Therapy Association (Alliance Communications Group)

Journal of Speech Language Hearing Research (American Speech-Language-Hearing Association)

Ostomy/Wound Management (Health Management Publication Inc.)

Physical Therapy: Journal of the American Physical Therapy Association (APTA)

PT Bulletin American Physical Therapy Association (APTA)

Rehab Management: The Interdisciplinary Journal of Rehabilitation (CurAnt Communications Inc.)

Home health practice is impacted by so many regulatory agencies, it is wise to become involved in a professional organization for home health providers. The National Association for Home Care maintains contact with federal legislators to keep up with any potential changes that could affect home health care and to express concerns on behalf of home health professionals. Participation in a home care organization is especially beneficial now that we are facing new financial challenges from managed health care payors, including Medicare. Along with the financial restraints, there are also additional demands in the forms of the Interim Payment System, Outcome and Assessment Information Set (OASIS), and a need for increased documentation to justify reimbursement.

Table 1-2	WEB SITE AND INTERNET RESOURCES FOR HOME CARE PROVIDERS

Agency for Health Care Policy & Research http://www.ahcpr.gov./guide
Alzheimer's Association http://www.alz.org/
American Cancer Society http://www.cancer.org/
American Diabetes Association http://www.diabetes.org/professional.htm
American Heart Association (AHA) http://www.amhrt.org/
American Nurses Association http:/www.ana.org/ or
    http://www.nursingworld.org
American Occupational Therapy Association http://www.aota.org/
Angels of Mercy http://www/aofm.com/
American Physical Therapy Association http://www/apta.org
American Speech-Language-Hearing Association http://www.asha.org
Arthritis Foundation http://www.arthritis.org/
Centers for Disease Control and Prevention (CDC) http://www.cdc.gov/
Health Care Financing Administration: The Medicare and Medicaid Agency
    http://www.hcfa.gov/
HIV Info Web http://www.infoweb.org/
Home Care Nurse http://junior.apk.net/~nurse/
Homecarequal listserv@listserv.medec.com
Homehlth listserv@list.iex.net
Hospice Foundation of America http://www.hospicefoundation.org/
Internet FDA http://www.fda.gov/fdahomepage.hltm
Intravenous Nurses Society http://www.insl.org/
Joint Commission on Accreditation of Health Care Organizations
    http://www.jcaho.org/
National Association for Home Care http://www.nahc.org/
National League for Nursing http://www/nln.org
Orthopaedic Section-American Physical Therapy Association
    http://www.orthopt.org
U.S. Department of Health and Human Services http://www.dhhs.gov/

Home health practitioners cannot become too complacent about their political responsibilities. They need to
remain current with state and federal legislation that affects home health practice. They need to provide input
to their congressional representatives on behalf of their
clients and the home health industry. When there is a
lack of input from the professionals, lawmakers may in-

stitute inappropriate standards. It is easier to influence standards before they are instituted than it is to get them changed later. It cannot be assumed that the legislators are knowledgable about the cost effectiveness of home health care or about the increased danger of rehospitalization or nursing home placement if home health care becomes unavailable. Legislators may not even be aware of all of the implications of their legislation unless we provide that input.

Following are some professional organizations that have been established to support the home health professional.

> American Occupational Therapy Association
> American Physical Therapy Association
> Association for the Advancement of Wound Care
> INS, Intravenous Nurses Society
> Home Healthcare Nurses Association
> National Association for Home Care

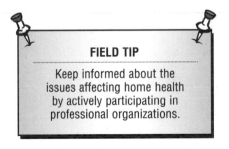

FIELD TIP

Keep informed about the issues affecting home health by actively participating in professional organizations.

References

Ceslowitz, S. B., Loreti, S. T.: Easing the Transition from Hospital Nursing to Home Care: A Research Study. Home Healthcare Nurse, 1991; 9(4):32–35.

Harris, M.: The Physician as a Member of the Home HealthCare Team. Home Healthcare Nurse, 1998; 16(11):732–735.

Hefty, L. V., Kenyon, V., Martaus, T., et al.: A Model Skills List for Orienting Nurses to Community Health Agencies. Public Health Nursing, 1992; 9(4):228–233.

Home Care 101: The Patient Controls the Home. Homecare Education Management, 1996; (1):1–3.

Gorski, L. A.: Case Management: Collaboration is Essential. Home Health FOCUS, 1998; 5(5):38.

Kenyon, V., Smith, E., Hefty, L. V., et al.: Clinical Competencies for Community Health Nursing. Public Health Nursing, 1990; 7(1): 33–39.

Martin, J. P.: Home Care Orientation Manual. California Association for Health Services at Home, Sacramento, 1995.

Narayan, M. C.: Survey Highlights the Concerns of Home Healthcare Nurses. Home Healthcare Nurse, 1999; 17(1):57.

Nicoll, L. H.: Nurses' Guide to the Internet, 2nd edition. Philadelphia, Lippincott, 1998.

Olsten Health Services: Transitional Nurses Orientation Learner Guide, p 10–2. Melville, NY, Olsten Health Services, 1997.

Sherry, D.: Time Management Strategies of the New Home Care Nurse. Home Healthcare Nurse, 1996; 14(9):718–720.

Snow, L., Hefty, L. V., Kenyon, V., et al.: Making the Fit: Orienting New Employees to Community Health Nursing Agencies. Public Health Nursing, 1992; 9(1):58–64.

Stoker, J.: The Regulatory Changes of 1998. Home Healthcare Nurse, 1998; 16(11):740.

Thobaben, M.: Understanding the Internet and World Wide Web. Home Care Provider, 1999; 4(4):10–12.

Transitioning to Home Care: Follow these 6 Tips to Orient Ex-hospital Nurses. Homecare Education Management, 1996; 1(1):1–3.

Yuan, J. R.: Using Standards and Guidelines in Your Daily Practice. Home Healthcare Nurse, 1998; 16(11):753–759.

Managed Care and Payor Sources

2

This chapter introduces you to the concept of managed care and all of the various types of third-party payors that are involved in managed care, which finances much of health care today. The discussion includes federal and state agencies, health maintenance organizations (HMOs), preferred provider organizations (PPOs), and other sources of private insurance. It also discusses different types of case managers and their roles in the delivery of health care. The chapter concludes with a discussion about some of the forms of regulatory compliance that affect home health practice.

Managed care employs principles of utilization management to maintain cost containment in health care. There is a great deal of public concern regarding the cost of medical care. Some of the techniques used to control and monitor costs are pre-admission, concurrent, and retrospective reviews by the various third-party payors.

ORIGINS OF MANAGED CARE ORGANIZATIONS

To understand the managed care organizations and their regulations with which the nurse or therapist must deal it is helpful to begin with a discussion of the origin of these agencies.

Some of the major organizations are agencies instituted by the federal government. As we learned in civics class, the legislative branch of the federal government passed the laws that established many of the agencies that regulate home care. The Social Security Act of 1935 and the Medicare Act of 1965 are two major legislative acts that form the basis for home care regulations.

FEDERAL GOVERNMENT AGENCIES

Table 2–1 lists the various agencies that originated in the federal government. The legislative branch writes and passes the laws that establish these various programs. The executive branch is responsible for enforcing the laws, which includes the implementation and administration of the programs mandated by these laws. The judicial branch interprets the laws governing these programs and reviews executive decisions concerning these laws.

Health and Human Services

The executive branch of the federal government is responsible for the administration of these acts. One of the departments of the executive branch is Health and Human Services (HHS). That department, which is organized into five principal operating components, administers many of the agencies that regulate home health. The five departments within Health and Human Services are the National Institutes of Health (NIH), Human Development Services, Health Care Financing Administration (HCFA), Social Security Administration (SSA), and Specialized Units of HHS.

The NIH includes the Food and Drug Administration (FDA), Health Resources and Services Administration,

Table 2–1 HEALTH CARE REGULATORY AGENCIES OF THE FEDERAL GOVERNMENT

LEGISLATIVE BRANCH Writes and passes laws	EXECUTIVE BRANCH Enforces laws			JUDICIAL BRANCH Interprets laws
	HEALTH AND HUMAN SERVICES			
→	→		→	→
→	→		→	→
National Institutes of Health	Human Development Services	Health Care Financing Administration (HCFA)	Social Security Administration	Specialized Units
→	⇊	→		→
• Food & Drug Adm. • Health Resources & Services • Substance Abuse & Mental Health Services • Centers for Disease Control	• Nutrition Programs • Head Start Programs	• Medicare • Medicaid		• Civil Rights • Child Support Enforcement • Consumer Affairs • Admin. on Aging (AAA)

Substance Abuse and Mental Health Administration, and the Centers for Disease Control (CDC). The Department of Human Development Services provides grants to the states to finance Nutrition Programs for the Elderly and Head Start Programs. The HCFA, established in 1977, regulates Medicare and Medicaid. The SSA, established in 1946, regulates the Social Security system. The Specialized Units of HHS include Civil Rights Administration, Child Support Enforcement, Consumer Affairs, and the Administration on Aging (AAA) which develops programs for older persons and provides grants to the 50 states and to Native American communities.

Health Care Financing Administration

The HCFA is the major regulator of home health reimbursement by Medicare. Many managed care organizations use HCFA regulations as a basis for their own regulations. Medicare is administered by HCFA, which contracts with some intermediaries to handle the reimbursement for Medicare services.

The intermediary is either a public or a private organization that is responsible for processing provider claims for Medicare service, auditing for unnecessary services, and communicating Medicare policy changes to the providers. There can be some variance in how the regulations are interpreted from one intermediary to another, but they all follow the same regulations. In the past, HCFA and the intermediaries were a little more relaxed with their interpretation of the regulations. Since the Balanced Budget Act of 1997, however, certified agencies are expected to adhere to the Medicare regulations more stringently.

Medicare

Medicare is divided into Part A and Part B. Part A pays for the hospital insurance, some home health care, and some days in a skilled nursing facility. Those who are eligible for Part A coverage need to have earned at least 40 quarters, which are determined by the number of years that the individual worked in the United States and paid into the Social Security system. Part B, a voluntary program, provides supplemental medical insurance. Clients' Medicare cards, indicate for which parts of Medicare they are eligible.

The SSA is responsible for overseeing the eligibility and enrollment of Medicare beneficiaries. Those eligible for Part A have the option to buy into Part B. If individuals do not take the option to obtain Part B coverage as soon as they become eligible for Medicare but decide to do it later, the fee to buy in is increased.

Some individuals who have not earned enough quarters (40 quarters) to be eligible for Part A can still buy into Part B. They will qualify for the same services as they would get from Part A. Examples of people who might fit into this category are legal immigrants who did not work for a sufficient number of years before retirement or a woman who did not work enough years before she retired and whose husband died before he had earned enough quarters.

Before the Balanced Budget Act of 1997, most of home health care was paid for under medicare Part A. Now Part A will finance post-institutional home health services for 100 days as long as:

> the home care is provided within 14 days of discharge and the client spent at least three days in an acute care or skilled nursing facility

If the aforementioned criteria are not met, benefits are paid under Part B.

If more than 100 days of home health care is required by the individual and the services continue to meet Medicare requirements, the services will then be paid for out of Part B. It is the intermediary's responsibility to keep track of the number of days for each client.

Medicare Part B also pays for certain durable medical equipment (DME) such as hospital beds and wheelchairs as long as there is a doctor's prescription for the equipment. Chapter 3, Medicare Conditions of Participation, reviews the regulations regarding DME in more detail. Part B pays for DME on an 80/20 basis. In other words, Medicare will pay for 80% of the equipment, and the client pays for 20% of the bill.

In addition to providing Medicare and Medicaid, HCFA performs some quality-focused activities, including regulation of laboratory testing, surveys, and certification and development of coverage policies. Any agency that performs laboratory procedures rather than sending them to an independent laboratory must follow the regulations covered by the Clinical Laboratory Improvement Act (CLIA) of 1988. This Act is a HCFA program that requires a laboratory registration certificate, depending on the type of tests that are performed.

Other federal agencies that directly affect your practice in home health are the FDA and the CDC. Nutrition programs for the elderly provide money for nutrition services, which may be an excellent resource for some of your clients. The Administration on Aging, one of the specialized units of HHS, provides money to assist clients with activities of daily living (ADL), nutrition services, respite care for caregivers, and housekeeping services that clients are not able to manage because of their illness.

Medicaid

Medicaid, which provides health insurance for the poor and disabled, is administered by the individual states but regulated by the federal government. The states set up contracts with home health agencies to provide services for clients who are eligible for Medicaid reimbursement.

Medicaid criteria have some similarities to Medicare criteria. The criteria require that services are provided by a Medicare-certified agency, there is a physician's plan of care for skilled or personal care, and prior authorization has been obtained. The Medicaid program will vary from state to state. Some states may have a waiver for the certified agency requirement, especially in areas where there may not be a certified agency.

Services covered by Medicaid also vary but could include visits made by registered or licensed practical nurses, home health aides, or personal care workers. The visits may be on an intermittent or shift basis. The shifts may last anywhere from 2 to 8 hours. Each state requires that the plan of care is updated on a regular basis.

The frequency of the updates varies. Many states require that the update take place every 62 days. In addition to nursing and personal care, other services that a state may cover under Medicaid are homemaker, respite, transportation, and meals on wheels.

Most states ensure that there are no other available payors for the client before declaring him/her eligible for Medicaid. Because of the variance of coverage from state to state, you need to become informed about the particular coverage in the state in which you practice. Refer to your agency's copy of the Licensed Agency Manual for this information.

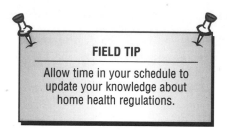

FIELD TIP

Allow time in your schedule to update your knowledge about home health regulations.

STATE GOVERNMENT AGENCIES

All agencies must be licensed by the state in which they operate. Just like the federal government, state governments are organized into three branches: the legislative, executive and judicial (Table 2–2). The executive is composed of the governor, other elected officials, and the heads of the state departments and agencies. Many of the department heads are appointed by the governor. Some of the departments found in each state are those concerned with education, police, public building programs, health and safety, and highways.

The home health agency must submit to unannounced surveys (i.e., audits plus visits) by the state. An agency must be licensed within the state in which it operates before it is eligible to become Medicare certified. Presently, the HCFA contracts with each state to perform a Medicare survey of certified agencies at the same time as the state survey is done.

On-site surveys occur when the license is first issued and when it is renewed. The state may choose to conduct surveys more frequently, especially if there has been a complaint against the agency. A home care agency that is certified to provide Medicare-reimbursable services is expected to remain compliant with the Civil Rights Act

| Table 2–2 | HEALTH CARE REGULATORY AGENCIES OF THE STATE GOVERNMENT |

LEGISLATIVE BRANCH (ASSEMBLY)	EXECUTIVE BRANCH (GOVERNOR)	JUDICIAL BRANCH (COURTS)
Writes and passes laws	Enforces laws	Interprets laws
	<u>Programs</u> Health Public Education Police and Safety Building Highways	
	<u>Departments</u> Economic Security Medicaid Nutrition Programs Health Services Professional Boards Councils of Government	

of 1964 and agrees to give Medicare beneficiaries the same services it provides to the general client population.

As most people understand, the Social Security system provides insurance for old age, survivors of workers, and those who are disabled. Coverage by Social Security does not automatically mean that an individual is eligible for Medicare coverage. For example, individuals are eligible for Social Security at age 62 years, but they are not eligible for Medicare until they reach the age of 65. Also an individual who is over age 65 but joins an HMO gives up Medicare benefits. Instead, Medicare pays the HMO a monthly fee to provide the client with health care. There can be variations concerning Medicare eligibility.

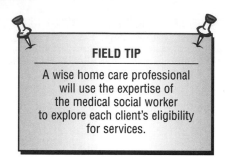

FIELD TIP

A wise home care professional will use the expertise of the medical social worker to explore each client's eligibility for services.

States also administer federal and state funds that provide resources to be used for additional services to benefit your clients. Some of those resources include assistance for the developmentally disabled and for families with dependent children. Other state departments that affect your practice as a home health professional are the department that licenses health care agencies within the state and all of the professional boards that license and regulate the practice of professionals in that state.

Each home health agency is expected to adhere to any regulations mandated by the local community in which it operates. The agency also is expected to adhere to its own policies and procedures. Surveyors will assess the agency's records to make sure that the agency is in compliance with all these regulations. Nurses and therapists are legally responsible for remaining up to date on federal, state, and local regulations and their own agency's policies and procedures. If the agency is penalized for noncompliance with regulations because of errors in your documentation, you could also be held responsible depending on the seriousness of the infraction. It will not do you any good to say that you did not know the regulations or that you did not have time to properly document the care provided.

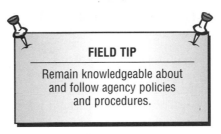

FIELD TIP

Remain knowledgeable about
and follow agency policies
and procedures.

As a case manager, you will find that Medicare is only
one payor that you will be dealing with when providing
client care. Many of the other payors have adopted some
of the Medicare regulations, but regulations vary from
one payor to another. The following discussions will review the various types of payors that you will be expected to work with in your everyday practice.

HEALTH MAINTENANCE ORGANIZATIONS

The basic premise on which HMOs were founded was
that clients would pay a monthly fee for the HMO to provide preventative care to keep them healthy. If a client required hospitalization or some other treatment because
of illness, the HMO would arrange for that medical care,
free of charge. Most of the original HMOs did operate
under these principles. As health care costs have risen,
HMOs have been restricting their coverage more. Now
they try to minimize the length of hospital stays and re-
strict usage to select providers. Usually the clients must
use certain facilities in the local area, which are serviced
by the HMO.

There are different types of HMOs. The staff HMOs hire
physicians to provide basic medical care to the members.
Frequently clients see a different doctor at each appointment. Many HMOs will assign, or have the member se-

lect, a primary care physician (PCP) who acts as a "gate-keeper" for ordering services.

Group HMOs contract with a group of physicians to provide medical services for their members. Independent Physician Association (IPA) HMOs contract with physicians or groups of physicians who have independent practices to provide the medical services. Some HMOs may be a combination of the above-described organizations. The more independent the physician, the more likely the client will have the opportunity to see the same doctor for their medical services.

In recent years, HMOs have redefined just how much medical care they will provide. Any care must be approved by the HMO before it is provided, except in the case of an emergency. When there is an emergency, there is no guarantee that the services will be paid. If the member happens to become ill when traveling outside the HMO's service area, the client will not be reimbursed for the care except if it is an emergency. For example, a member who needs elective surgery will be expected to travel back to the HMO's designated hospital for that procedure. Frequently, the client cannot purchase prescription medications outside the service area. The health care professional needs to make every effort to obtain approval for services from the HMO before those services are rendered.

If a Medicare client joins an HMO, the monthly fees are paid for by Medicare. Many clients and medical personnel do not understand that once clients join an HMO, they are no longer eligible for Medicare reimbursement. The HMOs are required to inform people of this regulation before they enroll, but many people miss the implications of this rule. They think that they can still use their Medicare as a secondary insurance. We need to remind them that they no longer have access to Medicare reimbursement as long as they are a member of an HMO.

The HMOs are required to provide the same basic services to their Medicare-eligible members as they would receive under Medicare. Encourage your clients who are considering joining an HMO to investigate thoroughly what is being offered and compare the benefits with what they already have. If clients are taking several medications, they might benefit by joining an HMO, but some other clients would probably be better off staying with Medicare. Lately, more and more HMOs are limiting the number of Medicare clients they enroll or are declining to enroll Medicare clients because HCFA has reduced the amount of money paid for each client. HMOs must give proper notice before "disenrolling" any members.

Usually, HMOs have certain times during which members can join or leave the HMO. The members also have the right to remove themselves from the HMO, but they must give proper notice, which is usually at least 30 days before the end of the enrollment period. When a home health nurse or therapist becomes aware that a client may be considering joining an HMO, the client should be reminded that she/he needs to inform all of the health care providers when the switch is made so the providers can obtain approval for the services from the HMO. If that does not happen, it is very likely that the services will not be reimbursed. Agencies can lose a lot of money when they discover too late that the client has switched payors and did not notify the providers. When admitting clients to the agency's services, make a point of explaining to them about the rules regarding HMOs, even if they are not members of one at the time and ask them to notify the agency if they should decide to join one.

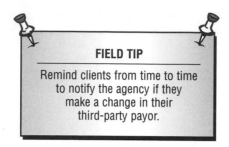

FIELD TIP

Remind clients from time to time to notify the agency if they make a change in their third-party payor.

PREFERRED PROVIDER ORGANIZATIONS

Preferred provider organizations (PPOs) are insurance organizations that provide their members with a list of various health care providers, including physicians, in-patient and out-patient facilities, and medical equipment companies. If the member selects a provider from the list, the insurance will pay for a higher percentage of the services than if the client selects a non-contracted provider. This type of program allows more flexibility for its members than an HMO. Some PPOs also assign primary care physicians to act as gatekeepers in an effort to contain health care costs.

PRIVATE INSURANCE

The home health nurse or therapist frequently cares for clients whose primary or secondary payor is a private insurance company, such as Blue Cross/Blue Shield. Insurances companies vary in how they operate and the amount of coverage they provide. Some have indemnity programs that cover a percentage of the cost of the care. Others have managed care programs in which they have established fixed-rate fees for particular services. Some insurance programs function as modified HMOs, whereas others function as PPOs. Others may offer both methods and allow the member to choose which one to use. Some insurance companies enter into contracting arrangements with certain providers to render services to their members in a particular community.

No matter what type of payor is providing the reimbursement, the health care provider needs to obtain prior approval for the services, except for Medicare. With Medicare, the provider needs to have an ongoing working knowledge of the conditions of participation that govern reimbursement. Prior approval is first obtained when the referral comes to the agency. The size of the agency and its method of organization determine who is responsible for obtaining the approvals. Larger agencies may have an admissions nurse who handles all of the referrals and obtains the initial approvals. In other offices, the clinical supervisor is responsible. In small offices, the professional case manager may be the one responsible for obtaining the approvals for care.

Each office needs to have the admission process clearly defined so everyone knows who is responsible for this function. The approval process is one responsibility that no one wants to slip through the cracks. An agency cannot afford to lose money because someone forgot to obtain prior approval for the visits. Frequently, the insurance company will approve an initial visit for evaluation and then expect the nurse or therapist to call for further approval of visits after the evaluation is completed.

Usually the approval will consist of a specific number of visits, such as four visits, depending on the client's primary diagnosis. The expectation is that the nurse or therapist will teach the client or a family member to perform needed procedures. It is surprising how quickly some lay people can learn to administer an intravenous antibiotic, but others run into problems that prevent them from learning the procedure within the allotted period of time. In those cases, the nurse or therapist needs to advocate for the client to obtain additional time.

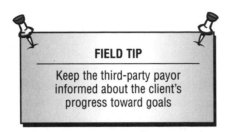

FIELD TIP

Keep the third-party payor informed about the client's progress toward goals

PRIVATE PAYMENT

Unlike Medicare and Medicaid, most other payors will not pay for aide services. Some clients and their families feel that it is more cost-effective for them to pay for aide services than to go into a skilled nursing or assisted living facility. Frequently a medical social worker will be used to assess the situation to see if there is another payor available to assist the client before she/he commits to private payment. Sometimes it might not even be necessary for the medical social worker to make a visit. The nurse or therapist might consult with him/her about available resources that can be explored to assist the client. Other services for which the client might be required to pay are medications, tube feedings, or housekeeping.

CASE MANAGEMENT

There are many different types of case managers involved in health care. When someone identifies himself or herself as a case manager, you need to get more information about his/her particular role. Some home health case managers are registered nurses or therapists who are responsible for coordinating the client's care and acting as an advocate for the client. Some case managers, who are usually registered nurses or social workers in an in-patient facility, are responsible for discharge planning and making arrangements for the actual discharge of the clients when they are ready to return home.

Another type of case manager is the individual who represents a third-party payor. These individuals may be registered nurses or social workers or they may be non-licensed and working under the supervision of a registered nurse or physician. Their focus may be on decreasing the length of service to control costs, but they also need to function as a client advocate. Some case managers, like those employed by an insurance company, provide telephone management, while others may provide varying degrees of on-site management.

Basically a third-party payor case manager is responsible for identifying high-risk and high-cost clients to assess their treatment options. The third-party case manager collaborates in the development of treatment plans while controlling costs, whereas the home health case manager needs to manage a client's total care to ensure an optimal outcome for the client.

It would be helpful to find out the background of the third-party payor's representative with whom you are communicating in order to acquire approval for visits to treat the client. This information will help you determine how much data the individual needs to make an informed decision. If you are not receiving satisfactory approval to assist the client, you might ask to speak with the representative's supervisor.

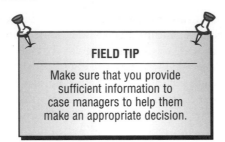

FIELD TIP

Make sure that you provide sufficient information to case managers to help them make an appropriate decision.

As a home care practitioner, you are responsible for managing the costs of care but you are also legally responsible that the client receives safe and effective health care. Presently, the health care agency, nurse, therapist, and physician are all held legally responsible for the client's health care; however, the insurance and managed care companies are not. Be sure to always document any conversations that you have with case managers, including their complete name, even if that communication results in a refusal to approve services. Include all the client information that you gave to justify the needed services. It is helpful if the nurse or therapist asks the case manager to send the refusal of services in writing. It's amazing how many case managers might reconsider the decision if they have to put it in writing with their signature.

REGULATORY COMPLIANCE

A home health agency is responsible for complying with regulations from many different agencies. There are some regulations that you use frequently and will probably always remember; however, each organization has its own set of regulations. Some of these regulations are similar to those of other agencies but others are different.

Each agency needs to have the written regulations from each regulatory institution available to the home care professional so information can be looked up when needed. Keep in mind that the different organizations update regulations from time to time, so you need to remain current with that information. Home health agencies need to make the revised regulations available to the field staff; additionally, the field staff needs to take advantage of that information. When you are dealing with an organization with which you are not familiar, you need to take the time to review the regulations that affect the care you are providing at that time.

If agency managers are smart, they will schedule reviews of the agency policies and procedures on a regular basis and perform quarterly chart audits as part of their quality assessment process. You might be expected to participate in the quality assessment process at your agency. Look on this participation as a learning opportunity. It has been found that newly hired professional staff members have improved their documentation skills after they participated in chart reviews.

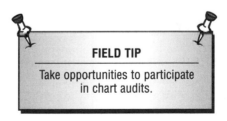

FIELD TIP

Take opportunities to participate in chart audits.

All professionals must have a working familiarity with the state practice acts that affect their disciplines. Each agency needs to monitor all of licensed personnel to ensure that they have current licenses. This requirement does not relieve individual professionals of the responsibility to make sure their licenses are current. The wise agency management will verify the licenses of newly hired personnel and of those current employees whose licenses are due for renewal.

Agencies must also remain in compliance with local community regulations including city and county ordinances. These usually are based on laws to protect the safety of the community. The requirements will include the need for a business license and enforcement of fire codes and proper disposal of hazardous waste.

Additionally, all professionals are legally responsible to be familiar with and follow the company policies and procedures. If legal action results because you are not following company policy and procedure, you will not be excused because you "did not know" it was against policy or you did not agree with the policy. Because of the varying regulators that affect home health there are bound to be discrepancies. If the regulations differ, the most stringent regulation should always be followed.

ACCREDITATION

Accreditation of an agency is usually a voluntary process. Most organizations realize the value of passing an accreditation process. The Community Health Accreditation Program (CHAP) and the Joint Commission on Accreditation of Health Care Organizations (JCAHO) accredit home health agencies. Accreditation implies commitment to quality, which involves submission to an objective, third-party review. The standards or criteria used to evaluate an organization are established based on input from home care providers and professional organizations.

When organizations are preparing for an accreditation survey, they find that they learn a great deal about how to provide high-quality care and service to the clients. The process pushes the agency staff to scrutinize their documents to make sure that everything is in compliance with all regulations. The process of preparation assists the organization in designing or refining its processes and procedures.

The accrediting organizations make sure that each agency is in compliance with not only the accrediting criteria but also with any required state and federal regulations. The fact that an agency is accredited promotes confidence in the staff by patients, physicians, and the general community. Potential employees value an agency that is accredited.

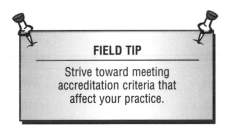

FIELD TIP

Strive toward meeting accreditation criteria that affect your practice.

References

Arizona Certified Agency Policy Manual: COP Interpretive Guidelines for Home Health Agencies, pp B–13 to B–20. Phoenix, Department of Health Services, 1997.

Benner, M.: The Medicare Interim Payment System's Impact on Home Health Services. Home Care Provider, 1998; 3(3):169–170.

1998 Grolier Multimedia Encyclopedia. Health and Human Services, US Department of. Danbury, CT, Grolier Interactive Inc, 1998.

1998 Grolier Multimedia Encyclopedia. Social and Welfare Services. Danbury, CT, Grolier Interactive Inc, 1998.

Hartley, W. and Vincent, W.: American Civics, 4th edition, pp. 43–45; pp. 122–129. Orlando, Harcourt Brace Jovanovich, 1983.

Medicare Bulletin #413, by bcc (Blue Cross California) Fiscal Intermediary, Oxnard, CA, January 15, 1998 p. 8.

Medicare Bulletin #416, by bcc (Blue Cross California) Fiscal Intermediary, Oxnard, CA, July 13, 1998 p. 13.

Olsten Health Services, Transitional Nurses Orientation Learner Guide, pp 7–1 to 7–14. Melville, NY, Olsten Health Services, 1997.

Popovich, M.: A Look Back at 10 Years of Home Care Accreditation at the Joint Commission. Home Care Provider, 1998; 3(6):326–328.

Popovich, M.: Why Become Accredited? Benefits and Values of Joint Commission Accreditation. Home Care Provider, 1998; 3(3):173–175.

Wellmark Fiscal Intermediary: Medicare Guide to Billing for HHAs, pp 1–22. Des Moines, IA, Wellmark, Inc, 1997.

Western Arizona Council of Governments: Area Agency on Aging Services Information Pamphlet, pp 6–9. Yuma, AZ, WACOG, 1997.

Medicare Conditions of Participation

3

The Health Care Financing Administration (HCFA), under the Department of Health and Human Services, is responsible for defining the Conditions of Participation (COP) for Medicare. The COPs are the requirements that home health agencies must follow to maintain their certification to provide services for Medicare reimbursement. The COPs lay the basis for home health practice.

This chapter discusses the COPs that affect the home health professional's practice and what that practitioner's responsibilities are in relation to these regulations. Since there are frequent changes in these regulations and their interpretations, space has been left on the right-hand margin for the reader to make updated notations.

The home health nurse or therapist must have a working knowledge of the COPs. The professional field staff have a responsibility for ensuring that these conditions are maintained, even though they are not responsible for the case management of the clients. The nurses and therapists are the ones who see the clients on a regular basis and are in the best position to know if their care remains in compliance with COPs. They are responsible for the assessment and evaluation of the clients to determine if they are eligible for Medicare home health services and if that eligibility is maintained. In addition, they need to know which services qualify for reimbursement and what documentation is necessary to demonstrate the client's continuing eligibility.

BASIC MEDICARE CRITERIA

Basically, the client who is eligible for Medicare benefits must be 65 years or older, have a valid Medicare card, be disabled, or have end-stage renal disease (ESRD). Disabled individuals must demonstrate a total and permanent disability for 24 consecutive months before they are eligible.

Medicare criteria for provision of home care include a Medicare-certified agency, reasonable and necessary services, homebound client, qualifying skilled services, a physician's plan of care, and services received in a place of residence. Table 3–1 lists the basic Medicare criteria required for reimbursement of services.

Certified Agency

A home health agency must move through a federal approval process to become certified by HCFA. This must be done before the agency can receive compensation for the care of Medicare-eligible clients. This process authorizes participation in the Medicare program.

The HCFA has delegated to state agencies the responsibility of determining whether home health agencies (HHAs) satisfy and continue

Table 3–1	MEDICARE ELIGIBILITY CRITERIA

Client 65 years or older, disabled, or with ESRD
Valid Medicare card
Certified agency
Reasonable and necessary services
Physician's plan of care (POC)
Homebound client
Skilled services
Services in place of residence

to satisfy the COPs in Medicare programs. In other words, the states not only initially determine the agency's eligibility by certification but reassess periodically the agency's continued compliance with Medicare's COP's.

Regional intermediaries, such as Blue Cross of California, have been designated by HCFA to process Medicare bills and make payments to the home health agencies. The intermediary is responsible for performing coverage compliance reviews to assure that services meet Medicare program requirements. The reviews also verify that the 485 information matches the client's medical record and claim. The 485 is an HCFA-designated form that each agency uses to record and certify each client's plan of care, as ordered and signed by the physician. A sample of the 485 form is included in Chapter 6, Client Admissions.

Reasonable and Necessary Services

The agency must provide reasonable and necessary services for the client experiencing an active medical, psychiatric, or surgical condition. It is usually an acute condition; if the illness is chronic, there must be evidence of recent exacerbation. The determination that services are reasonable and necessary is based on clinical documentation by the professional staff.

These services must be those that the client or family caregiver are unable to provide without assistance. (Either they do not have the skills or are not physically able to provide the care.) The nurse or therapist is responsible to determine if the client or caregiver is capable of learning how to provide the care. If after sufficient attempts to teach, the client or caregiver is not willing or able to be trained, further teaching would not be considered reasonable and necessary. It is expected that the duration of care by the agency will be temporary. In other words, the home health practitioner will work efficiently to help the client or caregiver learn to manage the necessary care.

The services provided for a particular condition must be consistent with that condition and its severity. Further, the services and their amount, frequency, and duration must be reasonable.

The identification of functional limitations can be used to indicate that skilled services are reasonable and necessary. Any one of four areas can be used to justify a functional limitation in a client.

The four functional limitation areas include: mobility, activities of daily living (ADL), communication, and safety.

Some conditions that indicate mobility limitation are limited ability to transfer or to ambulate. Examples of limited ADL are reduced ability to feed or dress oneself. Communication limits that could be used to justify service are difficulty swallowing or aphasia. Safety limits that could be used are a high risk for falling or lack of awareness of safety issues.

Physician's Plan of Care

The physician's plan of care (POC) must reflect that the client's medical needs demonstrate that the services are reasonable and necessary. It is expected that all pertinent diagnoses, the client's prognosis, rehabilitation potential, functional limitations, permitted activities, medications, treatments, and instructions for a timely discharge are included in the POC.

The POC must be signed and dated by a physician. The COPs define a physician as a doctor of medicine, osteopathy, or podiatry who is legally authorized to sign orders for the health care services provided. The orders must specify the disciplines needed to provide services, the frequency of visits, and the duration of the visits. (The duration of visits is the number of weeks required to help clients reach their goals.) Guidelines for determination of frequency and duration will be provided in Chapter 6, Client Admissions. Table 3–2 lists the elements that must be included in the POC.

Table 3–2	PLAN OF CARE REQUIREMENTS

All pertinent diagnoses
Client's prognosis
Client's mental status
Rehabilitation potential
Types of services, supplies, and equipment ordered
Functional limitations
Activities permitted
Nutritional requirements
Medications or treatments
Safety measures to protect against injury
Discharge plans

Any changes made in the POC must be ordered by the physician. For example if the frequency of visits by the nurse, therapist, or aide is increased or decreased, there must be a signed doctor's order. In addition, the doctor must be kept informed of any problems or changes in the client's condition. All of these communications must be reflected in the documentation. All orders must be signed by the physician prior to billing for the service. Discharge orders also must be signed by the doctor and on file in the client's record.

Homebound Client

The client must be homebound. Grasping the concept of homebound status is one of the biggest challenges facing the new home health professional. The HCFA is considering changing the definition of homebound by defining the number of hours per week or month that the client could be absent from the home and still be considered homebound. This change is being delayed until there are sufficient data to establish appropriate parameters.

Currently, Medicare's definition of homebound is "that status, due to illness or injury, that would require a considerable and taxing effort for the client to leave the home." The client who requires the aid of supportive devices, the use of special transportation, and/or assistance from another person could be designated as homebound. Another reason the client may be considered homebound is (if because of the medical condition) it is medically contraindicated for him/her to leave home.

The client does not have to be bedridden to be considered homebound but does have to be unable to leave home at will. The client who has undergone recent surgery, such as a total hip replacement, could meet the homebound requirement because of the risk for infection, even if the situation is temporary. A client with a psychiatric problem would be considered homebound if, because of the illness, she or he refuses to leave home or if it would be unsafe for him/her to leave unattended.

The client's environment can also affect the homebound status of the individual. For example the client might have to maneuver a flight of stairs or a steep incline, which interferes with his/her ability to leave home.

Clients who are able to leave the home could still be considered homebound if those absences are infrequent, for periods of relatively short duration or are to receive medical treatment. Basically there are three factors that help to determine if the client can be considered homebound.

1. The client is essentially confined to home
2. The confinement is related to a medical or physical condition
3. If the client does leave home, it is infrequently and/or for medical treatment, i.e., doctor's appointment.

See examples of qualifying and non-qualifying absences from the home in Table 3–3.

Table 3–3   QUALIFYING AND NON-QUALIFYING ABSENCES FROM HOME

QUALIFYING ABSENCES FROM HOME
Doctor's appointments
Kidney dialysis
Adult day care for medical treatment
Short or infrequent walk outside
Short or infrequent drive
Radiation therapy

NON-QUALIFYING ABSENCES FROM HOME
Playing cards with friends once a week
Adult day care for custodial care only
Senior activity center 5 times a week
Daily trip to McDonalds for coffee
Able to drive self to store or doctor's appointments
Walks around block without need for rest or assistance
Weekly trips to the mall

Clients who are able to leave home without assistance and get in and out of a car without assistance are *not* considered to be home-bound. Clients who walk with a walker and require assistance getting in and out of the car would be considered homebound. Examples for documentation of homebound status are provided in Chapter 4, Documentation.

Skilled Services

The next Medicare criterion is that there is need for skilled services. Skilled services can be provided by a nurse or therapist and must be reasonable and necessary for the treatment of the client's illness or injury. Skilled nursing can be provided by a registered nurse (RN) or, in some states, a licensed practical (vocational) nurse (LPN/LVN) under the supervision of an RN. The qualifying therapies include physical therapy (PT), occupational therapy (OT), and speech-language pathology (SLP) services.

A service is considered skilled when its complexity requires that it can be safely and effectively performed only by a skilled practitioner. Nursing, physical therapy, and speech therapy are primary skilled services, meaning they can admit clients for services. Occupational therapy and medical social services are secondary services, meaning that before they can be used, the client must be receiving one of the other skilled services. Once a client is receiving (OT) services, the client can continue to receive these services even if the other skilled services have been discharged, as long as the continued services are reasonable and necessary.

Qualified physical therapy assistants or occupational therapy assistants may provide services under the supervision of a physical or occupational therapist. The use of PT or OT assistants depends on the laws of the state in which the services are provided. Visits made by skilled professionals to train other agency staff are not billable services.

Maintenance therapy is a qualifying skilled service rendered by a PT, OT, or SLP. It becomes appropriate when repetitive services are required to maintain the client's level of function. Documentation needs to demonstrate that there is a high probability of regression (e.g., client with multiple sclerosis) and a need for a qualified therapist to manage the maintenance program.

Medical social services can be provided for a client who meets the basic Medicare criteria and qualifies for skilled services. Medical social service reimbursement tends to be more limited than other skilled services. It is expected that only a few (two or three) visits are necessary. The social services must be for a problem related to the client's current illness or injury, need for care, response to treatment, or adjustment to care. These services can include one furnished to a family member, on a short-term basis, when it can be demonstrated that the intervention removes an impediment to the effective treatment of the client. The medical social worker can be used if the client or family needs assistance to access community resources to obtain medications, housing, or medical supplies. If properly qualified, the social worker could provide counseling services to help the client adjust to the illness. The medical social worker cannot continue services when the client has been discharged by the nurse and the therapist.

Respiratory therapy (RT) services are allowable only as administrative costs to the agency. Visits by the RT are not billable separately. The services of a dietitian or nutritionist are also allowable only as administrative costs and are not billable separately.

The provision of home health aide services and durable medical equipment (DME) depends on the need for skilled services. In other words, Medicare will reimburse for aide services as long as there is a nurse or therapist providing skilled services. Once the nurse or therapist determines that the client has reached the goals or no longer qualifies for home care and is ready for discharge, the services of the nursing assistant are discontinued. Additionally, if skilled services by a therapist are placed on hold and they are the only skilled services provided, the services of the certified nursing assistant (CNA) are discontinued.

If there are indications that the client's current condition is long-standing and there are no attempts to resolve the condition, such as a client with chronic congestive heart failure or peripheral vascular disease, the skilled services would not be considered reasonable and necessary. Likewise, if after a reasonable period of time the client or caregiver is not willing or able to be trained to provide the services, further teaching would not be considered reasonable and necessary.

MEDICAL EQUIPMENT AND SUPPLIES

Medicare will reimburse for some medical supplies and durable medical equipment (DME), such as a wheelchair or hospital bed:

1. When skilled services are being provided in the home
2. Equipment is necessary and reasonable for treatment of the client's illness or injury or to improve functioning
3. Physician writes a prescription for the supplies or equipment.

Durable medical equipment is defined as equipment that can withstand repeated use, is primarily and customarily used to serve a medical purpose, is generally not useful in the absence of illness or injury, and is appropriate for use in the home. All elements of this definition must be met before the item can be considered to be durable medical equipment. DME is reimbursed under Medicare Part B.

Equipment is considered necessary when it contributes to the improvement of the client's condition or disability. Equipment is considered reasonable if

The expense of the item is proportionate to the therapeutic benefit

The cost is appropriate

The item is a realistically feasible alternate pattern of care

There is no equipment already available to the client that could essentially serve the same purpose.

Some equipment, such as oxygen equipment, is paid for on a rental basis. Medicare does not normally pay for the purchase of oxygen equipment. As with all equipment, documentation must indicate the medical necessity for use of home oxygen and equipment. The documentation needs to include:

A diagnosis usually thought to require O_2, e.g., chronic obstructive pulmonary disease (COPD)

Oxygen flow rate (2 L/min.)

Frequency and duration of use (lifetime necessity)

Client's pO_2 level.

There are some DME items for which Medicare will pay a monthly rental fee with a purchase option; these items are to exceed no more than 13 months of continuous use. If there is no purchase option, the monthly fee will be paid; however, the payment is not to exceed a period of continuous use of 15 months. Examples of DME and Non-DME are included in Table 3–4.

Medicare differentiates between routine and non-routine medical supplies. Medicare will

Table 3–4	DURABLE MEDICAL EQUIPMENT

DME
Wheelchair
Crutches
Hospital bed
Trapeze
Ventilator
Nebulizer
Commodes
Canes

NON-DME
Dressings
Catheters
Shower bench
Air conditioner
Incontinence pads
Physical fitness equipment
Self-help devices
First-aid equipment

reimburse for non-routine supplies that are needed to implement the POC for a specific client, such as supplies for a dressing change. Medicare will deny payment for any supply that's use is not documented. Routine supplies used for all clients, such as thermometer probe covers, are not billable. Non-DME and routine supply items, such as gel pads for clients with decubiti, are not usually reimbursed except if there is clearly a therapeutic purpose and they are reasonable and necessary for the treatment of the client's condition. Examples of routine and non-routine supplies are contained in Table 3–5. All services that could be covered by Medicare for reimbursement are listed in Table 3–6.

Table 3–5	ROUTINE AND NON-ROUTINE MEDICAL SUPPLIES

ROUTINE SUPPLIES
Alcohol preps
Non-sterile gloves
Thermometers
Masks
Tape removal pads
Tongue depressors
Probe covers

NON-ROUTINE SUPPLIES
Catheterization supplies
Dressing supplies
Syringes and needles
Intravenous tubing
Intravenous solution (without medication)
Slings
Tracheostomy care items

Intermittent Visits

All Medicare home visits, no matter which discipline is involved, are expected to be intermittent. This means that each visit usually takes from one to two hours; however there are exceptions. Usually the initial assessment

Table 3–6	SERVICES COVERED BY MEDICARE

Skilled nursing
Physical therapy
Speech-language pathology therapy
Occupational therapy
Medical social services
Home health aide services
Durable medical equipment (DME)
Non-routine medical supplies

visit will take approximately two hours. These time frames are not specified by Medicare, but are intended to provide guidelines for the practitioner who is new to home care. The visit length will vary on the basis of the client's needs and goals. Practitioners need to ensure that they are providing the time to which the client is entitled.

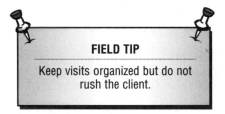

FIELD TIP

Keep visits organized but do not rush the client.

The definition of intermittent skilled care was clarified in the Balanced Budget Act of 1997. This clarification was an attempt to control abuse of Medicare but still provide flexibility to meet the varying needs of clients. The revised definition states the following criteria. Intermittent care is:

1. Provided or needed on fewer than seven days each week or
2. Fewer than eight hours of each day
3. For periods of 21 days or less
4. With extensions in exceptional circumstances when the need for additional care is justified.

The fourth criterion implies that exceptions need to be justified in the documentation and that a specific endpoint needs to be stated. Daily visits that extend beyond 21 days are visits that require careful documentation and a specific endpoint.

Administration of insulin is an example of a potential need for daily visits. The daily visits could continue for an extended period of time as long as:

Coverage criteria are met

Documentation shows that the client is mentally or physically unable to administer the injection

There is no willing or capable caregiver to administer the insulin

The client remains homebound.

A diabetic client who is blind and lives alone is an individual who could qualify for this extended service.

At the other end of the spectrum of visit frequencies is the need for infrequent yet intermittent skilled services. An example would be a client with an indwelling silicone catheter who needs a catheter change only every 90 days. Again the documentation needs to justify the frequency of visits.

The HCFA used to reimburse for venipunctures for laboratory tests; however, as of February 1, 1998, venipuncture is no longer considered a skilled service. Venipunctures can still be performed by the home health nurse as long as a qualified skill is provided during the visit, i.e., assessing or teaching. Table 3–7 provides a list of types of qualified nursing skills.

Table 3–7	TYPES OF QUALIFIED SKILLED NURSING

Skilled observation and evaluation
Teaching
Wound care
Injections
Catheter care
Dialysis
Intravenous therapy
Management and evaluation of care plan
Ostomy care
Psychiatric nursing

Management and Evaluation

Management and evaluation of a client's care plan can be an appropriate reimbursable skilled service. Situations that indicate a need for management and evaluation are characterized by client conditions or complications that require a registered nurse or physical therapist to ensure that the essential non-skilled care is achieving its therapeutic purpose. An aged client with a history of COPD and mild dementia who is recovering from pneumonia is an example of a client potentially in need of management and evaluation of the care plan. Since the client's age and medical and mental conditions indicate a high potential for complications, the management of the POC requires skilled services until the treatment regimen is stabilized.

Many health care professionals have problems understanding how to use management and evaluation appropriately, because of the complexity of its requirements. Some agencies do not even bother using the management and evaluation option as a skilled service because they do not understand it. There are some clients who's health would be jeopardized if they did not continue to receive care, e.g., a bedbound client, cared for by several family members.

To determine the need for management and evaluation of the POC, assess the client situation to determine if:

1. Inappropriate implementation of the care could put the client at risk for rehospitalization or exacerbation of the health condition
2. Care involves complex, unskilled therapy
3. Situation is unstable because of the changing nature of the POC or the individuals providing the care
4. Safe implementation of the plan requires the supervision of a registered nurse or therapist.

The client situation must meet all four of these criteria to qualify for management and evaluation. Examples of clients who could be at risk for rehospitalization or exacerbation are those who have multiple medical diagnoses or complications. An example of a client who could be at risk for admittance to an extended care facility, is one who, if the care is inappropriately implemented has a possibility of a decline in his/her function or loss of ADL skills. Since management and evaluation are considered skilled services, home health aide services can be used as long as they are reasonable and necessary.

The POC would be considered to constitute complex, unskilled therapy if there are many, complex medications and treatments or several resources required for the client's care. A caregiving situation that could be considered unstable is when several caregivers are involved in the care or if the only caregiver has a learning disability. Finally, a registered nurse or physical therapist is necessary to monitor the implementation of the plan to ensure safe care. All of the basic conditions of participation for Medicare, such as reasonable and necessary, still apply for coverage of a management and evaluation situation. Table 3–8 lists conditions or complications,

Table 3–8	EXAMPLES OF MANAGEMENT AND EVALUATION SITUATIONS

UNDERLYING CONDITIONS OR COMPLICATIONS
Multiple diagnoses
Chronic, complex, medical situation, e.g., AIDS
High probability of complications
Multiple or restrictive functional limitations
Defective mental status
Multiple rehospitalizations
Frequent exacerbations

COMPLEX UNSKILLED THERAPY
Multiple medications
Complex medical regimen
Multiple treatments
Multiple or complex pieces of equipment
Intense personal care requirements e.g., bedbound client

COMPLEX UNSTABLE CAREGIVERS
Multiple unskilled caregivers
Multiple community resources
Dysfunctional caregivers
Physical, mental, or cultural limitations of caregiver

Usually more than one item needs to be present to justify services.

complex services, and complex or unstable caregiving situations that could justify the use of management and evaluation services.

The case manager's (RN/RPT) primary responsibility is to supervise the POC and coordinate services required by the client. The case manager will also observe and assess the client's condition, but these responsibilities are secondary. Skilled management and evaluation require a specific doctor's order when it is the only skilled service rendered. Documentation for management and evaluation will be discussed in Chapter 4.

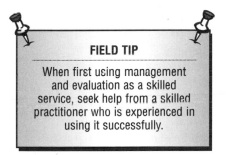

FIELD TIP

When first using management and evaluation as a skilled service, seek help from a skilled practitioner who is experienced in using it successfully.

Home Health Aide

Home Health Aide (HHA) services are used to provide hands-on personal care needed to maintain the client's health or facilitate treatment of the client's illness or injury. Home health aide services that qualify for reimbursement include personal care, simple dressing changes, assistance with medications that are ordinarily self-administered, assistance with activities that are supportive or extensions of skilled therapy, and routine care of prosthetic and orthotic devices. Nurse Practice Acts must be considered when preparing a care plan for the aide. For example, some states do not allow the aide to assist with administration of any medications. Other skills are allowed as long as the aide has had special training in the skill and has demonstrated competency in the performance of the skill to a registered nurse. Some states require that the aide demonstrate competency to carry out these special skills for each client who requires them.

During the home visit, the HHA may perform some incidental services that are not health related, such as light cleaning, meal preparation, or shopping. The purpose of the aide's visit may not be solely to perform these incidental services but must include personal services.

Table 3–9 provides examples of skills that fit the definition of personal care services. Table

Table 3–9	EXAMPLES OF PERSONAL CARE SERVICES

Bathing
Dressing
Hair care
Skin and nail care
Feeding
Assistance with elimination
Assistance with transfers and ambulation
Range of motion exercises
Incidental services, e.g., meal preparation

| Table 3–10 | EXAMPLES OF QUALIFIED PHYSICAL THERAPY SERVICES |

Evaluation
Teaching
Therapeutic exercises
Transfer training
Gait training
Prosthetic training
Whirlpool treatments
Wound care
Management and evaluation of patient care plan
Maintenance therapy program

3–10 lists examples of qualified physical therapy services; Table 3–11 lists qualified speech therapy services; Table 3–12 lists qualified occupational therapy services; and Table 3–13 lists qualified medical social services.

Medicare Exclusions

Some specific exclusions from Medicare coverage for home health services are drugs such as analgesics and biologicals, such as serums

| Table 3–11 | EXAMPLES OF QUALIFIED SPEECH THERAPY SERVICES |

Assessment and evaluation
Speech articulation disorder treatments
Dysphagia therapy
Language disorder treatments
Teaching
Prosthetic training
Restorative therapy
Maintenance program

Table 3–12	EXAMPLES OF QUALIFIED OCCUPATIONAL THERAPY SERVICES

Evaluation
Teaching
Activities of daily living (ADL) training
Muscle re-education
Fine motor coordination
Orthotics/splinting
Adaptive equipment
Cardiac rehabilitation exercise program
Plan and implement therapeutic program
Maintenance program

and vaccines. Transportation, hearing aids, and dentures are also excluded. Medicare Part B will reimburse for the pneumococcal pneumonia vaccine and the influenza virus vaccine and their administration.

STAFF QUALIFICATIONS

The COPs require that the agency be in compliance with regulations from all federal, state, and local departments that affect home health care. Each agency is also expected to always follow its own policies and procedures. The state and Medicare surveyors will

Table 3–13	EXAMPLES OF QUALIFIED MEDICAL SOCIAL SERVICES

Assessment of social and emotional factors
Counseling for long-range planning and decision making
Community resource planning
Short-term counseling for family or caregivers
Assessment of financial status

examine documentation and observe staff to make sure that the agency remains in compliance. The implication is that all staff members need to be aware of regulations, policies, and procedures that they are responsible for implementing. Further, the agency administration needs to assure that the staff members understand the various regulations, through in-service presentations. Sometimes the nurses or therapists may not realize the importance of following through on their responsibilities regarding these requirements.

The HCFA expects that the agency verifies the skills of each staff member hired. Each agency must identify exactly which skills, for each discipline, need to be verified before the practitioner can perform them independently in the field. It is expected that the individual verifying the skills can appropriately evaluate the skills of that particular discipline. For example, RNs observe RN, LPN/LVN, and CNA skills; and OTs observe other occupational therapists' skills. Additionally PTs observe other PTs and speech language pathologists observe other SLPs. A rare exception to this rule might be made in a small community agency that may have only one PT and one OT. Then the PT can observe the OT or vice versa.

The nursing assistant has several competencies to be verified. It may be most efficient to arrange to have the CNA observed while she/he is caring for some clients in a skilled nursing facility or transitional care unit. Another option is to have nurses make supervisory visits to observe the nursing assistant giving care in the home.

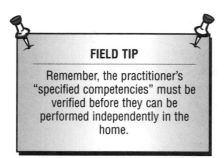

FIELD TIP

Remember, the practitioner's "specified competencies" must be verified before they can be performed independently in the home.

HCFA also requires that the field staff maintain their competencies through in-service sessions or continuing education. The number of required in-service sessions tends to vary according to state regulations. Nursing assistants are required by the Federal government to participate in at least 12 in-service hours per year. The agency is required to provide in-service training for the staff and to document exactly which in-service sessions and the number of hours attended by each individual. This documentation needs to be available on demand.

Lately, there is an increased concern by the general population that some abusive individuals are providing health care to vulnerable patients. To insure against this danger, states are beginning to require criminal background checks of home health care staff. Many home health agencies already perform background checks on newly hired employees but it is anticipated that in the near future all home health personnel will have to submit to background checks.

RECERTIFICATION

COPs require that each client's need for services be recertified every two months. Many clients will not require services beyond the two-month period but others will. At recertification time, the nurse and therapist who are still caring for the client must summarize the client's progress and determine if continued services are justified. If any of the skilled services are to be continued, the client must be reassessed, and a revised POC must be signed by the physician before the beginning of the next certification period. If there is a delay in receiving signed orders for the new certification period, interim orders must be obtained for any period of time not already covered by doctor's orders. Any visits that are not covered by doctor's orders will not be reimbursed by Medicare.

HCFA has indicated that they intend to become more stringent about holding nurses and therapists to the recorded, expected outcome dates for client goals. Up until now, HCFA has allowed more flexibility with those dates. In the past, some nurses and therapists got into the habit of using the end of the certification period as the expected outcome date. If the client reached the goals before that date, there was no problem. If they didn't reach the goals by that date, the professional would simply extend the outcome date to the end of the next certification period.

Medicare expects that when the documented outcome date is reached, the nurse or therapist will assess whether or not the goal was achieved. If the goal was not achieved, documentation must justify why the outcome date needs to be changed. Documentation must also explain what has occurred to delay achievement of the goal. If the client or family is not willing or able to learn how to provide the skill, however, the agency will be expected to discharge the client, and the client must seek some other alternative for care, such as a skilled nursing facility. This may sound controversial, but the rationale is that clients and families are expected to take responsibility for their medical care. Medicare is intended to be used to reimburse for home health services to help clients and families learn how to manage this responsibility, but it is not intended to be used to provide services for an indefinite period of time. Table 3–14 lists factors that determine the extent of Medicare coverage.

DUPLICATION OF SERVICES

Medicare will not cover services that are duplicated by other resources. For example, if the nurse is providing daily dressing changes but on one day the client sees the doctor, who changes the dressing during the office visit, the nurse should not make a home visit

Table 3–14	EXTENT OF COVERAGE

Visits predictable
Visits intermittent
Provided fewer than 7 days per week
For periods of 21 days or less
Endpoint required for daily visits
Extensions made in exceptional circumstances

(SKILLED NURSING AND HOME HEALTH AIDE COMBINED)
Up to 28 hours per week intermittent visits
Up to 8 hours per week intermittent visits
Or, Subject to review on case-by-case basis for care needed less than 8 hours per day and up to 35 hours per week

that day. Nursing and therapy should not be providing the same services, such as teaching the family how to provide range of motion exercises to the client. The nurse should not be providing any dialysis-related services when the client is receiving treatment at a dialysis center.

There may be occasions when the client requires services from two different agencies because one may not have the resources to provide all of the needed services, for example, if one agency does not provide PT or SLP services. Both agencies must be very careful that there is no duplication.

SKILLED VERSUS NON-SKILLED SERVICES

If the nurse is providing a non-skilled service such as a shower, it is still not considered a skilled service. In other words, the service is not considered "skilled" simply because it is performed by a nurse or therapist. On the other hand, an OT who assists clients shower to help them learn to care for themselves, would be providing a skilled service.

A skilled service still remains a skilled service even if it can be taught to a client or family member. If the family member who was originally taught the skill becomes incapacitated or unavailable, the nurse or therapist can resume care to teach another individual the skill. For example, a caregiver is taught how to administer an IV antibiotic but later has a cerebrovascular accident. Another family member can be taught the skill by the nurse or therapist.

PLACE OF RESIDENCE

Services must be provided in the client's place of residence. The place of residence is defined as wherever the client is residing. This may be his own home, an assisted living facility, or a home for the elderly. A place is *not* considered the client's residence if it meets the definition of a hospital or an extended care facility, i.e., a skilled nursing facility. If a residence such as an assisted living facility is licensed to provide care to the client (i.e., assistance with ADL), Medicare will not reimburse for like services, such as home health aide services but will pay for skilled services.

OUTCOME AND ASSESSMENT INFORMATION SET

Outcome and assessment information set (OASIS) is a set of data items developed by HCFA to be used to assess all clients served by a certified agency regardless of the payor, excluding maternal-child home care clients and housekeeping-only cases. The data items are used for measuring client-level outcomes of home care and for comparing outcomes between client groups. HCFA's model for measuring and comparing client outcomes using OASIS data is called outcome-based quality improvement (OBQI). The data items were developed as a result of a five-year national research program. OASIS is made up of 79 core items preceded by 10 routine identifiers.

The OASIS items are used by home health agencies to measure changes in client health and functional status over time. Measurements take place between two or more time points. The nurse or therapist is required to assess each client using the OASIS items at the following times:

Start of care (SOC)
Every two months (Recertification)
Discharge time
Transfer to an in-patient facility
Death of patient in the home
Resumption of home care.

Home care agencies will be required to transmit these data to HCFA on a monthly basis.

Transmission of data began August 25, 1999, for Medicare and Medicaid clients. Transmission of data for non-Medicare and non-Medicaid clients will begin in the spring of 2000. A client's admission data must be entered within seven days of the admission.

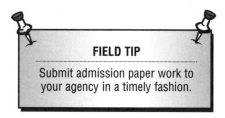

FIELD TIP

Submit admission paper work to your agency in a timely fashion.

It is expected that these data will provide an empiric basis for monitoring client outcomes by HCFA and each individual agency. HCFA will require each agency to select target outcomes to assess its own effectiveness with client care. Each agency will be expected to develop plans of action to overcome any deficiency that is demonstrated as a result of data analysis. More detailed discussion of the OASIS items will be addressed in Chapter 6, Client Admissions.

INTERIM PAYMENT SYSTEM

Under the Balanced Budget Act of 1997, the Interim Payment System (IPS) was established as a transition toward a prospective payment system. The prospective payment system is planned to be used for Medicare reimbursement of home health services. The intent of these systems is to place per beneficiary caps on the cost of home care. The prospective payment system will probably be based on particular client conditions or diagnoses. HCFA plans to use data collected under OASIS to develop the prospective payment system which, as of this writing, is predicted to come on line by October 2000. The home health industry is facing many new challenges with these changes in reimbursement. Individual agencies will need to learn to maintain a better case mix between short-term and long-term clients. They will need to educate clients, families, physicians, and other health care professionals about the proper use of home care services. Additionally, physician's need to be encouraged to inform clients and families about their responsibilities as a home health recipient.

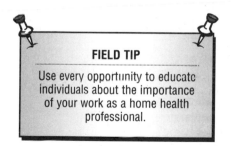

FIELD TIP

Use every opportunity to educate individuals about the importance of your work as a home health professional.

Nurses and therapists will be required to be even more accurate with client assessments and documentation. It will be crucial for more accurate determination of realistic client goals and expected outcome dates. The

IPS has created a serious financial impact on the home health industry. Several agencies have been forced to close. There are hopes that the prospective payment system will be easier for agencies to manage. Nurses and therapists need to remain informed about the effects of IPS on home health care and, when appropriate, keep their congressional representatives informed of any serious results.

The fiscal intermediaries (FI) have been required by HCFA to scrutinize the agencies' billing and related documentation more closely than before the enactment of the 1997 Balanced Budget Act. The FIs use certain criteria as guidelines to indicate potential abuses of Medicare reimbursement. If the FI determines that an agency meets one or more of these criteria, the agency will be required to submit to a focused medical review (FMR). This means that for a designated period of time, the FI will designate certain bills that will require the related documentation be sent for further review.

When agencies are notified of an FMR, they will be told what the percentage of their bills will be involved. The percentage is usually 25, 50, 75, or 100%. Each FMR will continue for a quarter, or three months. If the number of billing denials based on the documentation reviews exceeds a certain percentage for the quarter, the FMR will continue for another quarter. The agency does not know in advance which bills will be designated for the required documentation; that is done by the FI after the bills are received. FMR creates a great deal of time and expense on the part of the agency to meet the additional requirements. Thorough accurate documentation by the field staff members plays a crucial part in helping prevent FMRs for their agency or, if the agency is under a FMR, in helping the agency pass through one in a limited period of time.

Under the prospective payment system, the HCFA is expecting home health agencies to care for an increased number of low-cost beneficiaries, reduce the number of visits per client, and discharge clients earlier. Home care personnel will have to be even more diligent in the evaluation of the client's progress toward goals so the client is not kept on service any longer than necessary without jeopardizing the client's well-being. These changes may also mean that agency personnel will have to persevere in the education of physicians about the latest requirements.

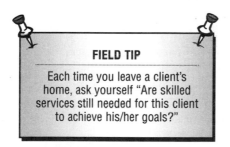

FIELD TIP

Each time you leave a client's home, ask yourself "Are skilled services still needed for this client to achieve his/her goals?"

Fifteen-Minute–Increment Billing

The 1997 Balanced Budget Act also requires that a code identifying the length of time for each visit, measured in 15-minute increments, be included on claims for home health services. This information is intended to be used for data collection. The HCFA defines the "time of service visit" to begin at the home, when delivery of services actually has begun. The timing includes in-home activities only. Two visits made on the same day are not to be combined as a single line item. Any services lasting fewer than 8 minutes are not reportable. The 15-minute increments will be reported as units. The units will be assigned as follows:

1 unit–8 to under 23 minutes
2 units–23 to under 38 minutes
3 units–38 to under 53 minutes, etc.

Providers are expected to deduct time interruptions for non-treatment related activities. This reporting has not been initiated at the time of this writing. The implications, if any, of this requirement to home health practice have not been fully realized at this point.

References

A Homecare Therapist's Guide to Medicare Service Delivery. The Beacon Homecare FOCUS Series. Medicare Reimbursement for Therapy Services, pp 1–9, Mequon, WI, Beacon Health, 1996.

Arizona Association for Home Care: Update: 15-minute Increment Reporting, March 12. Phoenix, AAHC, 1999.

Arizona Association for Home Care: OASIS Alert, June 18. Phoenix, AAHC, 1999.

Arizona Certified Agency Policy Manual: COP Interpretive Guidelines for Home Health Agencies, pp B-13 to B-20. Phoenix, Department of Health Services, 1997.

Benner, M.: Congress Approves Minimal Changes to Medicare Home Health Benefit. Home Care Provider, 1998; 3(6):312–313.

Benner, M. The Medicare Interim Payment System's Impact on Home Health Services. Home Care Provider, 1998; 3(3):169–170.

Can You Pass Home Healthcare Nurse's OASIS Quiz? Home Healthcare Nurse, 1999; 17(1):60–61.

Determining Homebound Status. The Beacon Homecare FOCUS Series, pp. 1–14, Mequon, WI, Beacon Health, 1996.

Hanneken, K.: OASIS Update. AAHC Arizona Homefront, 1998; 15(11):1.

Harris, M.: The Physician as a Member of the Home Healthcare Team. Home Healthcare Nurse, 1998; 16(11):732–735.

Health Care Financing Administration: BBA Implementation Tracking Report. Available at: http://www.hcfa.gov. Accessed February 11, 1999.

Health Care Financing Administration: Home Health Agency Manual (HIM-11) Chapter II, Coverage of Services, Sec 200, pp. 11–24. Washington, D.C., Department of Health and Human Services, 1987.

Health Care Financing Administration: Home Health Agency Manual (HIM-11) Chapter II, Coverage of Services, Sec 200, pp. 11–24. Washington, D.C., Department of Health and Human Services, 1996.

Health Care Financing Administration: Home Health Agency Manual (HIM-11) Chapter II Coverage of Service, Sec 234, pp. 11–24. Washington D.C., Department of Health and Human Services, 1998.

Hilliard, L. S.: Manager's Corner: Innovative or Disintegrate. Home Care Nurse News, 1998; 5(6):1–2, 8.

Hogue, E. The Behavioral offset of the Interim Payment System: What HCFA Expects Home Care Providers to do. Arizona Homefront, 1998; 15(6):10–11.

Management & Evaluation of a Care Plan. The Beacon Homecare FOCUS Series, 1996; pp. 1–16.

Medicare Bulletin # 416, by bcc (Blue Cross Calif.) Fiscal Intermediary, Oxnard, CA, July 13, 1998, pp. 13.

Medicare Reimbursement of Therapy Services. The Beacon Homecare FOCUS Series. pp.1–9, Mequon, WI, Beacon Health, 1996.

Milone-Nuzzo, P.: Beyond Venipuncture as the Qualifying Service for Medicare: Seeing the Forest for the Trees. Home Healthcare Nurse, 1998; 16(3):177–178.

National Association for Home Care: HIM-11 Coverage Guide for Field Staff. pp. 115–117, Washington, D.C., 1998.

Olsten Health Services: Continuing Nurses Education. Melville, NY, Olsten Health Services, 1996, pp 12–5 to 12–15.

Olsten Health Services: Training and Development, OHM/Introduction to Medicare SSG, 1/97. Melville, NY, Olsten Health Services, 1997, pp. 1-3 to 1-17, 3-3 to 3-4, 4-3 to 4-6.

Polzien, G., Kendall, B., and Hindelang, M: The challenge of implementing OASIS. Home Healthcare Nurse, 1998; 16(12):806–812.

Schroeder, B.: Medicare Case Management. Home Health FOCUS, 1998; 5(1):5.

Sitzman, K.: Tips for using OASIS. Home Healthcare Nurse, 1998; 16(8):561

Sperling, R.: How OASIS relates to the Medicare 485. Home Healthcare Nurse, 1999; 17(2):82–85.

Sperling, R.: What's this OASIS, Anyway? Home Healthcare Nurse, 1998; 16(6):373–374.

Stewart, M.: New Law Eases Medicare Interim Payment System Burden on Home Health Care. The American Nurse, 1998; Nov/Dec:10.

Stoker, J.: Defining Homebound Status. Home Healthcare Nurse, 1999; 17(2):119.

Stoker, J.: Home Care Voices Heard. Home Healthcare Nurse, 1999; 17(1):8.

Stoker, J.: OASIS as a Mandatory Medicare Requirement. Home Healthcare Nurse, 1998; 16(9):595

Stoker, J.: The Regulatory Changes of 1998. Home Healthcare Nurse, 1998; 16,(11):740.

Thomas, M. N.: Understanding Medicine Reimbursement. Home Healthcare Nurse, 1998; 16(12):840–843.

Wellmark Fiscal Intermediary: Medicare Guide to Billing for HHAs, Des Moines, IA, Wellmark, Inc, 1997 pp. 1–22.

Documentation 4

Documentation by nurses and therapists is always crucial but is even more critical in home health. Staff documentation has a direct effect on the results of billing for home care clients. Nurses and therapists are responsible for demonstrating, through documentation, the client's continuing eligibility for services. Home health agencies are in a unique situation because they have to produce the actual documentation when called for from the third-party payors. Home care is the only area in which billing is directly dependent on nursing and therapy documentation.

Another unique situation in home health is that there are usually only one or two individuals who are assessing the client (e.g., viewing the wound) on a regular basis. Accurate descriptions are important for keeping everyone responsible for the client's care informed about his or her progress. The readers for the various payors will be observing for consistency between the different staff members who are making chart entries about the same client. The more descriptive, measurable, and objective the charting; the better it is. Space is left on the right margin in this chapter to allow room for notes.

ELIGIBILITY FOR SERVICES

Documentation needs to reflect, on an ongoing basis, the client's eligibility for services including home bound status, need for reasonable and necessary services, skilled services received, and the client's progress toward goals. Home care agencies receive a great deal of scrutiny of client records from the various third-party payors and governments agencies that regulate home health.

BASIC DOCUMENTATION RULES

The same principles that govern documentation in hospitals and nursing homes govern documentation in home health. This book will not dwell on those basic principles but will focus on the differences found in home care. One major difference is that each visit note must stand on its own. Also, one must keep in mind that the initial payor reviewer may not be a health care professional. When documenting, you should never assume that the reader already has a complete picture of the client's condition.

Documentation of Wounds

When documenting a dressing change, you need to include a description of the procedure, including supplies used and a description of the wound. The following illustration demonstrates how this can be written:

Dressing change to right foot. Using aseptic technique wound packed with N/S soaked 4 × 4 s, covered with ABD dressing and wrapped with 3" gauze wrap and secured with paper tape. Wound 11 cm long, 15 cm wide, 1 1/2 cm deep. Surrounding skin reddened but cool to touch, wd beefy red, one 4 × 4 saturated with serosan-

guineous drainage, no odor, no s/s infection.
Socks and sheepskin boots applied.

....

In hospitals and other structured care facilities, merely stating that the dressing was changed and a description of the wound and drainage is sufficient. In home health, the nurse needs to document a thorough description of the wound and drainage at least once a week. The wound description needs to include measurements in centimeters of the length, width, and depth; its appearance; stage; drainage; and odor. There are individual paper tape rulers and plastic overlays that can be used to measure wounds.

Most agencies use skin assessment forms to screen and document the wound descriptions efficiently and accurately. Photographs of the wound provide an excellent means of documentation. The picture needs to be taken from the same distance each time, so the picture shows an accurate size. A 10-inch ribbon on the camera can be used to measure the camera's distance from the wound accurately and consistently. Since Medicare pays only for supplies that are actually used for the client, the visit note needs to list exactly which supplies were used during the visit. Document generic names for supplies rather than brand names, such as gauze wrap versus Kerlix. Medicare will usually reimburse for the least expensive brand, except if the more costly item can be justified as reasonable and necessary. The justification needs to be documented in the client's record.

Special Equipment

If special equipment needs to be used, such as an intravenous (IV) pump, its necessity must be documented. A nurse coming from an acute care facility may assume that everyone with an IV needs a pump, but not all third-party payors agree. Some examples for justification of a pump would be for the client who is receiving total parenteral nutrition or for a small child receiving IV fluids.

Most agencies have a set of approved abbreviations to be used for documentation. Be sure to use those abbreviations so the rest of the agency staff members understand what you are trying to communicate. Do not create new abbreviations just because it is easier for you. A list of abbreviations specific to home health are included in the inside cover.

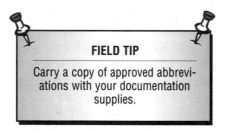

FIELD TIP

Carry a copy of approved abbreviations with your documentation supplies.

Make sure that your handwriting is legible. If it is not legible, you need to print your notes. Not only do you need to be concerned that personnel in your agency can read your writing, but you need to be concerned that reviewers from the payor sources can also read your writing, so they will approve the bill for your visit. If reviewers from the payor source have too much trouble reading the documentation, they may just deny payment of the bill.

Some agencies have portable computers for their nurses and therapists. These computers help the employees be more productive; employees do not need to worry about legibility of the handwriting. Other agencies use dictating machines and have notes typed by transcriptionists. The field staff needs to speak clearly when dictating to avoid mistakes in documentation.

THE VISIT NOTE

Documentation related to the initial assessment will be addressed in Chapter 6, Client Admissions. This chapter discusses the client progress notes that are made for the intermittent visits following the client's admission. There are certain factors that must be included in each visit note. Some basic factors that are generally included are client name, number, and signature; employee name and number; visit time; type of visit; and payor code.

Factors included in the body of the note are:

Vital signs
Physical and mental assessment data related to the plan of care
Skilled services provided and client response

Reason client is homebound
Instructions given
Progress toward client goals
Changes in client condition
Any changes in the plan of care
Plan for the next visit
Any physician contact.

Most agencies require that the client's signature be obtained at each visit to verify that the visit did occur. Unfortunately, this verification is required because payors have been billed for fraudulent visits in the home care industry. As in all health care documentation, the employee signs all visit notes.

Any documentation of time on the visit note needs to be accurate. If your appointment with the client is for 10 AM but you arrive at 10:10, you need to put 10:10 AM as your arrival time. Travel time and mileage are completed in the same manner. The actual time spent with the client helps to verify that the visits are part-time and intermittent. The times should not be rounded off. It is such practices that make auditors suspicious of fraud. Auditors also compare one employee's time and mileage with another's when they are traveling to the same client's home. It appears highly suspicious when an employee claims that she or he took 30 minutes to travel 5 miles. Never predate or backdate any documentation.

The type of visit needs to be recorded, because it helps determine whether the agency will receive reimbursement and for how much. Usually Medicare and other payors reimburse the same amount for an initial assessment as they do for a regular intermittent visit, even though the initial assessment takes more visit time and more documentation. To receive reimbursement for that initial visit, the documentation needs to demonstrate that an approved skill was performed. If the initial visit is for evaluation only, it will not be reimbursed.

Medicare does not reimburse for supervisory visits of aides or LPNs, although it is expected that they are being done. If the supervisory visit is combined with a skilled intermittent visit, it will be reimbursed. Required documentation for supervisory visits will be discussed in Chapter 8, Case Manager Responsibilities.

Some clients have more than one payor. Medicare may be paying for intermittent visits for IV therapy while Medicaid may be paying for aide services that require supervisory visits. The home care practitioner must be sure to document the appropriate code for the type of visit that is being made.

When making an intermittent visit, it is expected that the nurse performs a head-to-toe assessment. You are expected to focus your assessent documentation on client needs related to the plan of care. In other words, the care delivery is prioritized according to the plan of care.

If you are monitoring the client's vital signs or blood sugar level, the plan of care needs to

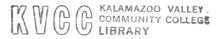

contain parameters, ordered by the physician, that will indicate at which point the doctor needs to be notified.

Visits should be documented on the same day of the visit. It is best to document during the visit rather than saving it until later. By doing so, your charting will be more accurate and efficient. Frequently, clients will take an interest in the documentation and add to the pertinent data. You will tend to remember questions that need to be asked better and will contribute to the documentation more effectively.

Some personnel prefer to document later. If you do choose not to chart during the visit, do not put it off too long. Many employees chart in their car immediately following the visit. Of course, that type of charting will depend on how safe you are in the neighborhood. If you put off all of your charting until the end of the day or, even worse until the next day, it takes longer to sort out the necessary data for each client, and it is easy to forget to record pertinent data.

Your documentation should be organized according to the plan of care and, more specifically, according to the client's goals. Each goal needs to be addressed at least one time each week. This is the rationale for developing realistic and measurable goals.

Any skills performed during the visit need to be documented clearly. Keep in mind that one of the Medicare intermediaries may be viewing the record. One item that they will be looking for are what skilled services were provided. Do not assume that they can interpret your documentation and surmise from it that you did perform some skills. Explain the required skills clearly. Reinforce the documentation by listing the skills that were administered, e.g., dressing change, peripheral vascular assessment.

Keep in mind which skills are reimbursable by Medicare (see Chapter 3). There are some skills that you would consider as being skills of your discipline but that are not reimbursable. Venipuncture is such a skill. It used to be reimbursed, but as of February 1998, that is no longer the case. Medicare would still reimburse for a visit in which you perform a venipuncture as long as you also document a reimbursable skill, such as skilled observation. If the payor for the visit happens to be different than Medicare, you need to become familiar with what skills are approved by that payor.

HOMEBOUND STATUS

Another factor that the fiscal intermediary will be looking for is documentation of the client's homebound status. Homebound status needs to be documented at least once each week. You may find it easier to include a homebound statement with each visit note.

If you happen to chart a statement indicating that the client is absent from the home, be sure the statement is clear that the absence is for a legitimate reason. Of course, if it is not an acceptable absence, it may be an indication that it is time to discharge the client. If

you are documenting that you have attempted a visit but did not receive a response
when you rang the door bell, describe it as:
*Rang door bell twice, knocked on door. No re-
sponse.* Rather than: Client not at home. The
client could be home but not able to get to
the door. Table 4–1 provides some examples
of statements that support homebound status for the client.

Table 4–1	STATEMENTS TO DOCUMENT HOMEBOUND STATUS

Ambulates 30 feet with walker and one assist.
Requires supervision due to confusion.
Unable to climb stairs; client lives on third floor.
Requires rest after ambulating 20 feet.
Severe pain limits ambulation to 25 feet in the home.
Bedbound due to generalized weakness.
Tolerates sitting up in chair no more than 30 minutes.
Requires assist of two to transfer from bed to chair.
Partial weight bearing. Must use walker to ambulate.
Requires assist of two to transfer from wheelchair to car.
Impaired vision. Requires one assist to leave home.
Must keep feet elevated because of open draining wounds.
Risk of infection because of open draining wounds.
Wheelchair bound. Unable to ambulate.
Dyspnea with minimal exertion. Must rest every 3 to 4
steps.
Requires use of walls and furniture to ambulate because
of unsteady gait.
Unstable blood sugar levels prevent client from leaving
home without supervision until control of diabetes.
Requires continuous oxygen. Not able to maneuver
equipment without assistance.
Phobic disorder prevents client from leaving home.
Disruptive behavior requires supervision of client when
leaving home.

Reasonable and Necessary Services

Your documentation needs to continue to demonstrate that the services provided are reasonable and necessary. Therefore, the services need to relate to the client's medical condition. For example if the client's only diagnosis is diabetes mellitus but you document that the only skill performed for the visit was administration of a Vitamin B_{12} injection, the visit will not be reimbursed. Another example is when the client's primary diagnosis is epistaxis and physical therapy is ordered. Either the wrong primary diagnosis was designated or it is inappropriate for the client to receive PT services.

Make sure that your documentation provides a description of the client's situation. Therapists need to keep in mind that the first reviewer of a third-party payor will probably not be another therapist. Avoid using abbreviations that are not generally recognized by a nontherapist. As you are charting, anticipate questions that the reviewers may have as they are reading the information. Such as when describing the client's functional limitations, go a step further to explain what specific activities the limitations are preventing. For example, you may document: *Client has generalized weakness.* But explain how that affects the client's activity: *Therefore, is unable to sit up for more than 30 minutes at a time.* Documentation of the client's functional improvement or lack of improvement related to therapy must be included.

The visit note also needs to indicate that there is a continuing need of skilled services. Medicare will not pay for services for a client with a chronic disease if the documentation indicates that the condition is stable. It is important to update the dates of exacerbation of the condition. Be cautious about using terms in your charting that indicate stability of the client's condition, if that isn't the situation. You need to keep describing the client and his/her medical condition. Such terms as *condition stable, looks better, feeling better,* or *no change in status* do not give a clear picture and may give the impression that the client no longer requires services.

Remember always to return to your basic principles of documentation: Do not state your opinion; describe what you are observing. That also goes for statements such as *uncooperative* or *noncompliant*. If you find that you are describing a client whose condition is remaining stable or who is not making any progress, it may be an indication that it is time to discharge the client.

Be sure to read over your charting before submitting it to the agency. Sometimes we are in too much of a hurry and end up documenting some embarrassing statements. For example: *A head to nose assessment was performed,* or *she tripped and fell while lying in bed.* Table 4–2 contains suggestions for documenting reasonable and necessary services.

FIELD TIP

Review your visit notes before submission. Do they document a skilled service, homebound status, and reasonable and necessary services?

| Table 4–2 | REASONABLE AND NECESSARY SERVICES DOCUMENTATION |

Pain: intensity, type, location, pattern, how relieved, effect on client

Gait Training: type of gait deviation, functional problems, amount of assistance needed, distance walked, client understanding

Wounds: stage, length, width, depth, skin color or condition, temperature, appearance, color, drainage, odor

Dressing Change: exact procedure, supplies and how used, how secured

Intravenous Therapy: type, size and site of needle, fluid, rate, solution, medications, rate, type of pump if used, site condition and care

Cardiopulmonary Assessments: capillary refill, pulses, apical pulse, edema, lung auscultation, nail beds, respirations, activity tolerance, color, skin temperature, pain, cough, sputum amount and color, sensation, oxygen, medications

Diabetic Assessment: blood sugar level, edema, numbness, skin lesions, peripheral vascular, appetite, diet, insulin, eye sight, orientation

ADL Training: level of function, level of assistance, exercises or activities, client performance, client understanding

Communication Training: functional ability, level of communication, client progress, exercises or activities

Progress Toward Goals

As previously stated, each of the client's goals needs to be addressed at least once a week in the documentation. The assessment and skilled observations should demonstrate objective measurable data relating to the client's goals. The visit note must include how the client is progressing toward each goal. There should also be an indication when any goal has been achieved. Keep in mind that once you document that a goal is resolved, it is expected that the goal will not be readdressed in the future unless there is a change in circumstances, e.g., the client develops a complication. Because of this, be sure that the client has actually achieved the goal before documenting that it has been reached. Table 4–3 provides some examples of proper documentation of a client's progress toward goals.

Teaching

Teaching is a skilled service that is an expected, on-going need of the client and family caregiver. Each visit note should contain documentation of teaching. The exception would be if you are visiting the client more than one time a day, e.g., when providing twice a day dressing changes; even then, however, there will probably be a need for teaching each time.

When documenting teaching sessions, indicate who received the instruction, such as client and/or spouse, and the subjects taught.

Table 4-3	PROGRESS TOWARD GOALS

Wound granulation increasing, no s/s infection.

Gait stability improved.

Progress in bed to wheelchair; transfers with one assist.

Gradual increase in weight gain/loss.

Fatigues easily.

Continues to be wheelchair-bound.

Continues to require continuous 2-liter oxygen.

Slow steady progress with learning diabetic care.

Requires verbal cues when performing self dressing changes.

Increased dependent edema (2+).

Episodes of chest pain continue 1 to 2 times per week.

Difficulty sleeping due to pain level.

No s/s infection at IV site.

Spouse beginning to learn to administer tube feeding.

Client continues total dependence on insulin administration because of blindness.

Client continues to require close supervision with administration of IV antibiotic.

Client continues to require walker and 1 assist for safe ambulation.

Also include how the client and caregiver demonstrated understanding of the content and how much understanding the individual demonstrated.

Example #1: Instructions given to client and spouse. Subjects taught: diet management, elevate feet. Client verbalizes food groups on the exchange list. Kept feet elevated on stool during visit.

Example #2: Demonstrated dressing change to daughter. Daughter gave a return demonstration. Required verbal cues throughout procedure.

Also include the teaching plan for the next visit. Such as: *Continue diet and foot care instruction,* or *Observe daughter's dressing change technique next visit.* Keep in mind that once your documentation indicates that learning of a certain subject is complete, there should be no reason to readdress the subject. So make sure that the learning is complete before you document that it has occurred. Also be mindful that you can't continue to teach a subject forever. When teaching a particular subject over an extended period of time, you must be able to demonstrate progress toward the teaching goal.

Change in Client Condition

Documentation needs to indicate if there has been a change in the client's condition. If so, was the physician contacted and what was the result of that contact? Was there a change or modification in the plan of care? If so, did the client participate in the planning of care. It is hoped that the client and caregiver will always have an opportunity to participate in the care plan.

Plan for Next Visit

Finally, you need to indicate your plan for the next visit. The intermediary will expect that at least one time during the client's care, the discharge plan is documented. There also needs to be documentation that the client or caregiver has been informed about the discharge plan at least one time prior to the actual discharge. With managed care, discharge planning should begin at the time of admission. You will find that the client will be better prepared when discharge actually occurs if discharge planning begins promptly. Table 4–4 provides some examples of statements used to indicate the plan for next visit.

MANAGEMENT AND EVALUATION

Chapter 3 includes a description of Management and Evaluation skills. Medicare recognizes that conditions could exist in the home that could lead to a setback, an accident, or inadequate treatment for the client. These situations require evaluation, coordination, and management of the plan of care by a registered nurse or therapist. Some client situations may be considered appropriate for management and evaluation during the initial certification period or later when the initial skilled care is no longer necessary. However, management and evaluation services are not appropriate if the only services needed are aide services or to simply monitor the client's condition to detect early signs of complications.

Table 4–4	PLAN FOR NEXT VISIT

Continue dressing change bid.
Discuss discharge plan with client/spouse.
Continue cardiopulmonary assessment weekly.
Teach s/s hypo- and hyperglycemia.
Review procedure for IV antibiotic therapy.
Observe dressing change procedure by caregiver.
Discharge next visit.

Ongoing documentation supporting management and evaluation is crucial when this is the justification for continued care. This documentation must begin with the initial assessment. Each visit note must reflect clearly the necessary skills provided and support why the skills could be provided only by a registered nurse or therapist, i.e., teaching and monitoring the provision of range of motion exercises. Each note should include client assessment data indicating risk and safety concerns, all skills including family caregiver and client education, counseling and supervision activities, and community resources that are used by the client. If a home health aide is required for the client's care, documentation also needs to justify that the aide's services are reasonable and necessary. In addition to recording the continued rationale for management and evaluation, documentation of communication with other staff members and the physician needs to be recorded.

As in any visit note, you need to include the client's response to treatment and his/her progress toward goals. Be sure to include any exacerbation of the client's condition. You need to focus on how the skills being provided are maintaining the client or caregiver's ability to provide the safe and effective care called for in the plan of care. For each visit, you need to document exactly what is being prevented by management and evaluation of the plan of care. This can be charted along with the client's progress toward goals or when documenting the plan for the next visit. Table 4–5 contains samples of statements that can be used to justify continuing management and evaluation services.

OTHER SITUATIONS

When the client requires daily or twice a day visits, the visit notes need to clearly reflect why the client continues to need such frequent visits. About the only situations that can justify daily or more frequent visits for short periods of time are for dressing changes, intravenous therapy, whirlpool treatments, or exercises for total knee replacement. The expectation is that if the skill needs to continue for an extended period of time, the client or caregiver should be taught to take over the provision of that treatment. If there is no one willing or able to provide the care, the reason needs to be documented on a regular basis.

Table 4–5	STATEMENT TO SUPPORT MANAGEMENT AND EVALUATION OF PLAN OF CARE

Client requires continued observation and education to prevent recurrence of episodes of pneumonia and rehospitalization.

Need for skilled nursing for assessment, teaching, medicine management to prevent further diabetic foot ulcers and rehospitalization to allow client to remain safely in own home, and avoid skilled nursing facility placement.

Skilled nursing need to assess and evaluate self-feeding ability to prevent aspiration when daughter absent from home.

Bedbound CVA client with episodes of confusion requires skilled therapy to supervise and assess non-skilled care by three members of family so client able to remain in residence.

Some reasons that would justify continued treatment by the nurse or therapist are: a client who lives alone and is blind or has arthritis; has a spouse who has Alzheimer's disease; or who has a spouse who is wheelchair-bound or terminally ill.

When an "as needed" (PRN) visit is called for, the visit note needs to reflect that it is PRN and why it was necessary. Keep in mind that all PRN visits must be covered by a physician's order. Remember to include all of the routine documentation, such as client assessment based on client goals, skills performed including teaching, client response to the care, and plan for the next visit. The typical types of visit that would require a PRN visit are to reinsert a Foley catheter or to restart an intravenous line.

CASE COMMUNICATION NOTES

All case communications must be documented. This includes communications with the physician, other team members, and any case managers from other resource agencies. Be sure to record attempted contacts as well as actual contacts. This documentation could prove valuable for reference purposes. Include changes in client condition, observations or problems, and contacts to obtain new orders. Any change in doctor's orders must be documented, dated, and include the physician's signature. If the doctor fails to date the orders, the agency needs to stamp the date on the orders when they are returned to the office. If the signed orders re-

Table 4–6	Documentation Tips

Use action words, e.g., instruct or evaluate.
Use measurable, objective data.
Be specific.
Be clear and concise.
Write legibly.
Focus on client's illness or disability.
Address each of the client's goals.
Avoid use of terms such as stable or WNL (within normal limits).

NEGATES MEDICAL NECESSITY
Avoid words such as "noncompliant," "uncooperative," or "refuses."
Use "difficulty following instructions."
Avoid "progressing well or improving."

main undated, any visits covered by those orders will not be reimbursed. Additionally, record any refusals for orders from the doctor or refusal for approval of treatment by the third-party payor. Table 4–6 contains some basic documentation tips.

Chapter 6, Client Admissions, contains documentation examples that can be used for the initial assessment and admission of the client to the agency services. That chapter also includes discussion of the various elements of the client's plan of care.

References

A Homecare Therapist Guide to Medicare Service Delivery. The Beacon Homecare FOCUS Series, pp. 1–9. Mequon, WI, Beacon Health, Medicare Reimbursement for Therapy Services, 1996.
Blanchard, L., Gill, G., and Williams, E.: Guidelines and Documenta-

tion Requirements for Social Workers in Home Health Care. Silver Spring, MD: National Association of Social Workers, 1991, Chapters 3 and 8.

Determining Homebound Status. The Beacon Homecare FOCUS Series. pp 1–14. Mequon, WI, Beacon Health, 1996.

Health Care Financing Administration: Home Health Agency Manual (HIM-11), Chapter II Coverage of Services, Sec 200, pp 11–24. Washington, D.C., Department of Health and Human Services. 1987.

Health Care Financing Administration: Home Health Agency Manual (HIM-11) Chapter II Coverage of Services, Sec 200, pp. 11–24. Washington, D.C., Department of Health and Human Services. 1996.

Health Care Financing Administration: Home Health Agency Manual (HIM-11). Chapter II Coverage of Services, Sec 234, pp. 11–24. Washington, D.C., Department of Health and Human Services. 1998.

Hogue, E.: The Behavioral Offset of the Interim Payment System: What HCFA Expects Home Care Providers to do. Arizona Homefront, 1998;15(6): 10–11.

Management and Evaluation of a Care Plan. The Beacon Homecare FOCUS Series. pp. 1–16. Mequon, WI, Beacon Health, 1996.

Medicare Reimbursement of Therapy Services. The Beacon Homecare FOCUS Series. pp. 1–9. Mequon, WI, Beacon Health, 1996.

Olsten Health Services: Client Care Management for Hospital Alliance Home Health Agencies. Documentation protocols. pp. 4–1 to 4–9. Tampa, FL, Olsten Management Services, 1995.

Schroeder, B.: Medicare Case Management. Home Health FOCUS, 1998; 5(1):5.

Stoker, J.: Defining Homebound Status. Home Healthcare Nurse, 1999; 17(2):119.

Wellmark Fiscal Intermediary: Medicare Guide to Billing for HHAs, pp 1–22. Des Moines, IA, Wellmark, Inc, 1997.

Infection Control

5

This chapter deals with standard (universal) precautions and medical asepsis as they relate to home care. This discussion includes the principles of bag technique and how they can be implemented.

Infection control practices in home health date back to the early home health agencies. Before the use of antibiotic therapy, precautions were taken to prevent the transmission of organisms from one home to another. Newspapers were widely used as barriers. Handwashing was practiced as the major means to provide infection control. Handwashing continues to be the single most effective means to prevent the spread of infection.

With the advent of antibiotic therapy, health care providers became more complacent with infection control practices. Although infection control practices were emphasized, because of the belief that antibiotics could handle any infection, people became more careless. Penicillin was the miracle drug for a short period of time, but soon we discovered that we had to keep increasing the dosage to achieve the same results. Then we had to find other antibiotics to control infections. Today we realize that antibiotics are not going to make up for our carelessness when practicing medical asepsis.

We are becoming more conscientious about handwashing. In home care, we have realized the need to return to the use of barriers and the bag technique. It is amazing how we keep having to learn the same lessons. Not only do we need to be concerned about carrying infectious organisms from one client to another but also about exposing ourselves and our family members to those same organisms. The possibility of this exposure is of special concern since most home care employees use their own vehicles when making client visits.

National infection control guidelines that are specific for home care still need to be developed. Presently, the guidelines developed for hospitals have been adapted for home care. Practitioners generally regard home care as a safer health-care setting because of the client's reduced exposure to infection from other clients and multiple caregivers.

STANDARD PRECAUTIONS

The Centers for Disease Control and Prevention (CDC) is the governmental organization responsible for identifying, preventing, and recommending treatment for communicable, vector-borne, and occupational disease in the United States. The CDC has recently released new regulations for infection control, called Standard Precautions. Standard Precautions combine the practices of universal precautions, used to reduce the risk of transmission of blood-borne pathogens, and body substance isolation, used to reduce the risk of transmission of pathogens from moist body substances.

Whereas universal precautions specified certain body fluids for which handling precautions were necessary, Standard Precautions consider all body fluids to be suspect. Standard Precautions require the use of protective gloves to guard against any potential contact with any body fluids except perspiration. A major difference is that Standard Precautions call for the use of precautions whether or not the body fluid contains visible blood. The primary blood-borne virus infections that we are concerned about preventing with Standard Precautions are those caused by hepatitis B (HBV), hepatitis C (HCV), and human immunodeficiency virus (HIV).

Personal Protective Equipment

The Occupational Safety and Health Administration (OSHA) requires home health agencies to supply all employees who are at risk for exposure to body fluids with personal protective equipment (PPE). This equipment includes gloves, body fluid–proof gowns and aprons, masks, eyeshields, and resuscitative equipment (CPR one-way valve). All home health personnel who come in contact with clients are expected to carry the personal protective equipment with them when making home visits. Surveyors will check to be sure that home care field staff are carrying their protective equipment.

Additionally, employers are required to train employees in the proper use of their personal protective equipment. The employer is responsible for maintaining proficiency with Standard Precaution practices by the employees. This training of newly hired and current employees must be documented by the agency. The documentation must include that each employee understands the basic content of the training. The training must at least include what PPE is necessary and when and how to use it properly.

Bag Technique

Next to handwashing, bag technique is the second most important means used by home health personal to control the transmission of infections. The clean section of the bag is reserved for any equipment that is directly used on the client, such as the blood pressure cuff and stethoscope. The basic principle of bag technique is that you never enter the clean portion of the bag without washing your hands. The implication is that handwashing materials and barriers must be carried in a separate section from the clean equipment.

When entering the client's home, locate an area to place the bag. Remember you are in the client's home so ask permission to use the area. Some homes are very cluttered. You may have to negotiate with the client and family to provide an area for the field staff to place their bags. Never place the bag on the floor, which is considered to be the dirtiest area. There are some homes in which, because of sanitation concerns, there is no place where you would feel comfortable placing the bag. In such an instance, place the necessary items in a clean plastic bag to carry into the home.

Once you find an area in which to place the bag, lay down a barrier and then place the bag on the barrier. The best barrier material is plastic so no liquids can soak through to the bag or equipment. Plastic grocery bags provide excellent barriers. They are free, and most people have many of them stuffed in a drawer at home. You can cut them open to provide a larger surface area or if you do not want to bother, two bags provide an adequate work area. Other materials that can be used as barriers are plastic wastebasket liners or paper towels. The barrier cannot be reused. If your barrier is not a plastic material, be careful not to place it on a damp surface.

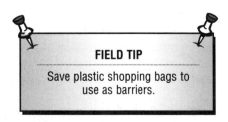

FIELD TIP

Save plastic shopping bags to use as barriers.

Supplies commonly carried by home health field staff in their bag include the following:

Paper Towels and Antibacterial Liquid Soap: You don't want to use the client's supplies. Many if them are on fixed incomes and frequently need to choose between buying meat or medications. Additionally, OSHA requires that employers provide each employee with hand-washing equipment. These items, along with barriers, are carried in an outer compartment of the bag for easy access.

Waterless Hand Cleansing Solution: Can be used as a substitute for soap and water. Up to ten applications can be used before you need to wash with soap and water. You will probably want to wash with soap and water much sooner, since hands tend to feel grubby after a couple of uses. This product does come in handy when you are in an area with no running water or when it is inconvenient to run to a sink. An example is when you are changing a dressing. When the soiled dressing is removed, you would like to wash your hands but not leave the open wound unprotected. The waterless cleansing solution can be used without leaving the client's side. Another occasion might be when you discover that you forgot to remove all of the needed equipment from your bag. Rather than returning to the sink, you can simply use some of the cleansing solution. The recommendation is to at least wash your hands with soap and water at the beginning and the end of the visit.

Bottle of 70% Alcohol with Sprayer: This is used to disinfect nondisposable equipment that is used to provide care from one client to another. It is easier to spray sphygmomanometers and stethoscopes than to try to clean them with alcohol wipes. Take care not to spray the plastic cover of the blood pressure cuff dial for it will cloud the plastic. Any equipment or supplies that have been taken out of the clean section of the bag must be disinfected before they are put back in the bag. Some home health staff put a supply of items such as universal precaution gloves in a baggie which is carried in the clean section of the bag. The baggie can be taken out of the bag and left on the barrier to be accessible when needed. If you do not use all of them on that visit, you can spray the outside of the baggie without damaging the gloves and replace it in the bag.

Thermometer Probe Covers: Used to cover thermometers for standard precaution purposes. Probe covers are especially susceptible to damage from extreme heat. They should not be left in a hot car, even for a short period of time.

Alcohol Wipes: For general use.

Standard Precaution Gloves: For standard precaution purposes.

Personal Protection Equipment: Required for standard precautions.

Routine Equipment: Equipment routinely used for each visit, such as thermometer, stethoscope, and sphygmomanometer.

Miscellaneous: Other supplies needed depending on the client goals, such as supplies for a venipuncture.

When the bag is not in use, it should be kept in a secure area. If the bag is stored in the car, keep it out of sight, preferably locked in the trunk of the car. If the bag is stored at home, it should be kept closed and out of reach of other family members. Each field staff member is responsible for the cleanliness of the bag. A bag should be cleaned out at least once each month. State surveyors have been known to inspect the bags of the field staff.

Another item that we carry from home to home is our clipboard or notebook containing our paper supplies. Most home health personnel have found that the type of clipboard in which you can enclose the paper supplies works well for home visits. For confidentiality purposes, only carry in paperwork related to the client's care; do not take in any information about another client. Frequently, you may use your clipboard for the client to write on when signing the visit note; therefore, you need to find a way of disinfecting it before you make a visit to another client's home. If your papers are enclosed within the clipboard, you can simply spray the outside with alcohol. If you are unable to protect your papers from the spray, you can wipe the underside with an alcohol swab. You could use a barrier for the clipboard but that tends to be awkward.

When preparing to leave the client's home, cleanse your hands. Then spray any items that you intend to return to the clean area of the bag. After packing the bag, wash your hands with soap and water. While washing your hands, also wash the outside of the liquid soap bottle. If there are any paper towels remaining, leave them for the client or family if they want them, otherwise dispose of them. Pick up your bag. Pick up the used barriers, handling them on the top side and dispose of them in the client's wastebasket.

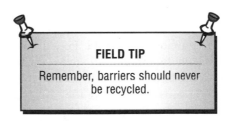

FIELD TIP

Remember, barriers should never
be recycled.

BIOHAZARDOUS MATERIALS

Any items containing body wastes need to be disposed of carefully. Items that potentially contain body wastes should be handled accordingly such as linens, clothing, sharps, diapers, dressings, and tissues. Find out the local regulations for biohazardous waste disposal. Wear gloves whenever handling these materials. Food and drink should never be kept in the same area where blood or other potentially infectious materials are found. Procedures involving blood or other body fluids should be performed to minimize splashing, spraying, spattering, and generation of droplets of these substances. If there is a potential for splashing, wear goggles. Glasses are not a substitute for goggles.

The disposable materials, such as diapers, dressings, and tissues, must be double bagged in plastic bags and placed directly into the client's trash bin outside. It should not be left in the home to expose the client's family to the infectious organisms.

Dispose of sharps in a puncture-proof container that is properly sealed before disposal. Most agencies provide containers for disposal of the employees' sharps. Blood samples for laboratory work must be placed in containers and labeled as biohazard. The specimens must be placed in a container that prevents leakage and labeled or color-coded to indicate that it is biohazardous. If there is a danger that the primary container has been or could be contaminated, it needs to be placed in a secondary container.

Soiled linen and clothing should be handled separately from other family linens. Do not shake linens since you can spread germs into the air. Dispose of the body substances into the toilet. Then have the caregiver wash the clothing and linens separately with soap and water.

CLIENT AND FAMILY EDUCATION

Home care agencies are caring for more acutely ill patients and providing more highly technical skills in the home than occurred 10 to 15 years ago. Since home care provides intermittent care, infection control standards of care still must be followed by the client and caregiver in the absence of the home care personnel.

A crucial step to ensure an effective infection control program in the home is client and family education. Begin by teaching the importance of handwashing and personal hygiene. Do not assume that clients and family members understand its importance. Observe how they wash their hands. Some people just rinse their hands off and consider them clean. Review with them the times when they should be washing their hands.

Provide guidance for when they should be using universal precaution gloves. Teach them how to dispose of diapers and dressings properly. Instruct them how to handle soiled linens. Encourage them to provide good ventilation throughout the home to prevent the spread of germs through the air.

Have them keep an appropriate container handy for disposal of sharps. The container needs to be made of aluminum or a hard plastic. Orange juice or milk bottles are made of a soft plastic that can be punctured by a sharp. A fabric softener or liquid detergent bottle is made of a heavier plastic that is puncture proof. Instruct them to seal the container before disposing of it into the trash.

Help the client and family caregiver learn to clean up body substances properly. They should be encouraged to wear latex or utility gloves and to use paper towels to wipe up spills and dispose of them in a plastic bag, which should be sealed before disposal. Then clean the area with hot water and soap. Apply a bleach solution made up of 1 part bleach to 10 parts water (1/4 cup bleach to 2 1/2 cups water). Remind them never to mix the bleach with other cleaning products, since dangerous fumes may result. The bleach solution will lose its strength after 24 hours, so it needs to be made up fresh with each use.

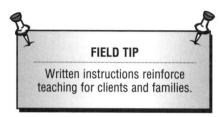

FIELD TIP

Written instructions reinforce teaching for clients and families.

Emphasize the importance of a clean work area that is free of dust and, if possible, away from household traffic. Keep work surfaces, equipment, and supplies disinfected. The work surface can be kept clean with soap and water. If disinfection is needed, 70% alcohol or a 1:10 bleach solution can be used to wipe the surface. Pets need to be kept away from the work area.

The client and family members need to learn that the client, because of his/her illness, is more susceptible to infections. Therefore, some practices, such as sharing personal items, that did not lead to infections before the illness could now cause a serious infection. They need to use clean dishes and utensils. Family members and visitors with a cold or flu must stay away. A cold in a normally healthy individual can mean pneumonia and sometimes death in a vulnerable client. Home health personnel need to remember this when they may be tempted to work with a cold or another contagious infection.

Clients and family members should be encouraged to take advantage of influenza vaccines except when it is medically contraindicated. Many physicians will recommend that the client also receive an immunization for pneumonia.

Client Education for Special Procedures

Intravenous Therapy: The Intravenous Nursing Society provides guidelines for intravenous (IV) therapy that can be used for teaching the client and caregiver. Areas of instruction that should be included in relation to infection control are: site care, sterile technique, and signs and symptoms of infection. Common practices to prevent infection include changing the dressing every 48 to 72 hours or when the integrity is compromised and changing tubing every 24 to 48 hours.

Meticulous care and aseptic technique are essential when one is caring for a central venous access device. The site should be inspected and dressed at least every 72 hours. Teach the client or caregiver to cover the site with an impermeable material when the client is showering or swimming to avoid exposure to potential organisms in the water.

Urinary Catheter Systems: Clean technique is considered adequate for intermittent catheterization in the home situation. It is more cost-effective for the client to use a reusable catheter for intermittent therapy. Teach the client to disinfect the catheter after each use. First, it should be washed with soap and water and then it should be boiled in water for 15 minutes. A pan and lid should be set aside to be used for this procedure only. Instead of boiling the catheter, it could be placed in a glass jar of water and heated in the microwave on high for 15 minutes. After boiling, the catheter should be dried thoroughly and stored in a closed plastic bag, clean towel, or clean dry jar with a lid. It should be kept in a clean, dry place. The inner lumen of the catheter can be dried by forcing air through it with a clean bulb syringe.

Clients with an indwelling catheter should be taught to cleanse the perineal area with soap and water on a daily basis and after each stool. Have them cleanse the catheter, wiping away from the meatus and stabilizing the tube so it does not pull out. The drainage bag should be cleaned and disinfected weekly. First rinse it with water then instill a white vinegar solution (1 part vinegar: 3 parts water). A poultry baster, purchased for this procedure only, can be used to cleanse the tubing. Another solution that could be used instead of vinegar is a bleach solution (1 teaspoon bleach to 1 pint of water).

Home Respiratory Care: It is not unusual for home care clients to require instruction about tracheotomy care. Sterile technique is required for new tracheotomies but for a tracheotomy that is more than a month old, clean technique is acceptable. Reusable suction catheters can be cleaned with soapy water, rinsed and boiled for 20 minutes. Plastic catheters can be flushed with sterile water and placed in 3% hydrogen peroxide. These should be flushed with sterile water prior to use.

Implanted Devices: Sterile technique must be used at all times when accessing an implanted devise until the area is healed. Emphasize handwashing, sterile technique, and observing for signs and symptoms of infection.

Enteral Feed Devices: Clean technique is appropriate for clients who are given tube feedings. Instruct the client and caregiver to avoid contamination of feeding solutions, which usually occur after the container has been opened. Commercial feeding solutions should be used within 24 hours after opening and must be kept refrigerated between feedings. The solutions need to be warmed to room temperature prior to feeding. The same principles apply for homemade feedings. Raw eggs should not be used to make homemade feeding solutions. The feeding bag and tubing should be rinsed with tap water after each administration. Feeding systems should be checked daily for damage and mold or fungus.

Dialysis: Medical asepsis is always crucial when dialysis is performed in the home. Sterile technique is always practiced when performing the procedure. The clients and caregivers must practice universal blood and body fluid precautions. They need to learn the signs and symptoms of infection, including the significance of a return of cloudy solute in peritoneal dialysis.

Wound Care: Client and caregiver education for wound care needs to include indications for handwashing and clean versus sterile technique. Also signs and symptoms of wound infections need to be emphasized. Proper storage and maintenance of supplies is indicated. Wound care protocols are going to vary according to the type of wound and physician preference. Fresh surgical and deep open wounds call for sterile technique. In the home, clean technique may suffice for superficial wounds as long as the physician agrees.

The home care professional is responsible to access the home situation for safety and appropriateness for care. The safety factors should include a consideration for protection against infection. Is there poor sanitation or rodent and insect infestation? Is there lack of appropriate infection control by the client or family caregiver?

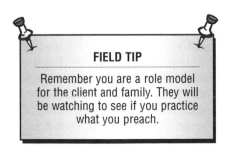

FIELD TIP

Remember you are a role model for the client and family. They will be watching to see if you practice what you preach.

OCCUPATIONAL EXPOSURE TO BLOOD-BORNE PATHOGENS

In 1989, OSHA published regulations regarding occupational exposure to blood-borne pathogens by health care workers. Today we are well aware of the dangers of exposure to hepatitis and HIV. We know that we must protect ourselves from exposure through use of standard precaution practices. Basic infection control practices usually are sufficient to prevent the transmission of blood-borne pathogens. Data show that in most cases of exposure, the practitioner was not practicing the basic precautions. Even when we are careful, accidents still can happen.

The employer is required to make the hepatitis B vaccine available to all employees who have occupational exposure to blood or other potentially infectious body fluids. Notice this involves all employees with occupational exposure, not just health care workers. If an employee initially declines the vaccination but later decides to have it, the employer is responsible to provide the vaccine at no cost to the employee.

When an exposure incident such as a puncture or splash occurs, it must be reported immediately after the exposed area has been washed. Needle-stick injuries constitute the major number of reported occupational exposures. The employer is responsible to provide post-exposure evaluation and follow-up for employees who have had an exposure incident, at no cost to the employees. The employer must ensure that the medical evaluation information is kept confidential.

The employer will identify the source individual whose body fluids were involved in the exposure. The employer is responsible for attempting to obtain permission from the source individual to determine his/her HBV and HIV infection status. If the source individual is known to be infected with HBV, HCV, or HIV, testing of his/her blood is not repeated. The results of the testing shall be made available to the exposed employee.

The exposed employee's blood will be collected as soon as feasible and tested after the consent is obtained. Within 15 days of the completion of the health care worker's post-exposure evaluation, the employer will obtain a copy of the evaluation and provide it to the employee. Documentation needs to include that the employee has been informed of the results of the evaluation and any medical conditions resulting from the exposure that require further evaluation or treatment. Follow-up HIV testing of the exposed employee is done at 6 weeks, 3 months, and 6 months if the initial test result is negative.

TUBERCULOSIS

Tuberculosis (TB) is becoming more prevalent today than it has been in many years. It is not likely that the client with active TB will be treated at home, but occasionally that could be the situation. On such occasions, the employer is responsible for providing properly fitted respirators for any employees who are involved in the client's care.

There is always a danger of the home health employee coming in contact with an individual with active tuberculosis. CDC guidelines indicate that the employer should provide medical surveillance, at no cost to the employees, for early detection of TB in employees who may have occupational exposure to TB. Any newly discovered case of TB must be reported immediately to the public health department.

Each agency is expected to have an active, effective infection control program. The employee is responsible for being familiar with that infection control program and maintaining compliance with it. For example, the employee should cooperate with the annual TB skin test program and make use of the personal protective equipment at the appropriate times.

The agency's infection control program begins with identifying infections in the client and employee populations. The agency depends on the home care professional to report any new incidences of infection. These data are examined to detect trends and problems. The nurses and therapists are not only responsible for following the infection control policies and procedures themselves but also for ensuring that the CNAs and LPNs that they are supervising are following the same policies and procedures. The infection control program should be part of the agency's quality improvement program.

REPORTABLE DISEASES

The CDC requires that state health departments report cases of selected diseases. The health care professional must be aware of and follow this requirement. Some of the reportable diseases include measles, AIDS, hepatitis, and TB. The local health department is the appropriate resource for questions about this requirement.

References

About Standard Precautions, pp 1–15. Deerfield, MA, Channing L. Bete Co., 1997.

About Infection Control in the Home, pp 1–15. Deerfield, MA, Channing L. Bete Co., 1995.

Epley, D. and Faria, S. H.: Assessment of Infections in Home Care Patients. Home Care Provider, 1999; 4(1):13–16.

Keating, S. B.: Infection Control in the Home Setting. Home Care Provider, 1999; 4(1):4.

Neighbors, M. and Monahan, F. D.: A Practical Guide to Medical-Surgical Nursing in the Home, pp 668–672. Philadelphia, W.B. Saunders Co, 1998.

Nelson, S.: The Importance of an Infection Control Program in Home Care. Arizona Homefront, 1999; 16(2):5.

Popovich, M. L.: The Joint Commission's Home Care Standards for Infection Control. Home Care Provider, 1999; 4(1):40–41.

Sommer, B.: Protecting our Patients and Ourselves. Home Care Provider, 1999; 4(1):30 33.

Wilson, T. H.: OSHA Guide for Health Care Facilities, Sec 513, 523, Appendix I. Washington, D.C., Occupational Safety and Health Administration, 1998.

Client Admissions

6

This chapter discusses the essential elements of the initial visit to assess the client for admission to agency services. It will include the importance of each element and suggestions for organizing the visit to make the best use of the client and nurse or therapist's time.

INTAKE OF ADMISSIONS

Each agency has its own specific system for handling client referrals. There may be a designated individual who initially handles all of the referrals. The responsibility may be shared by the clinical supervisors or it may be the responsibility of all the nurses and therapists that work for the agency. No matter what the basic procedure, everyone should be familiar with the necessary information that needs to be obtained when the client is referred.

Basic information obtained at the time of referral includes the client's name, address, residence phone, and another phone number if available. It is important that the address is accurate. If the referral is not coming from within the local community, be especially careful to obtain the correct address. There is nothing more frustrating for the nurse or therapist than to be hunting for a street name that is misspelled. Directions to the home would be helpful, but usually the referring agent does not have access to that information.

The referral information also needs to include the date of the referral and the expected start of care date. Most agencies try to begin care within 24 hours of the time of the referral or the time of discharge from the referring facility. If care does not begin promptly, it is important to document why there was a delay. If you are not the admitting professional but your services are ordered after the start of care, the 24-hour rule will usually still apply. Again, it is important to document any variances from the agency policies.

Other information needed by the admitting nurse or therapist includes the client's date of birth, client number, social security number, primary doctor's name, primary and secondary diagnoses, surgical procedures, and primary and secondary payors. Of course, you need to obtain the initial orders from the primary doctor. The doctor who writes the orders needs to be authorized to do so in the state in which the services are being provided; however, the doctor does not have to be located in the same community as the agency service area. Additionally, state regulations vary as to whether the attending physician must be licensed in the state in which services are provided. The home health practitioner must be familiar with these state requirements.

The nurse or therapist can make an initial assessment of the client to make sure she/he is eligible for home care services before obtaining doctor's orders, but in most cases it is more efficient to seek the orders beforehand. If there are no doctor's orders, the visit needs to be for evaluation only, and no skilled care can be rendered.

If the primary payor is not Medicare, it is wise to obtain written approval for home care visits from the appropriate third-party payor before the client is seen. That written approval can be in the form of a faxed message. If Medicare is the primary payor, the admitting nurse or therapist needs to make the initial evaluation to be sure the client qualifies for Medicare reimbursement. Although the client's eligibility will be evaluated during the initial visit, the one initiating the intake process can save everyone time by making the initial determination as to whether the home health agency is the appropriate provider.

PREPARATION FOR INITIAL VISIT

Once the nurse or therapist receives the referral information, she/he needs to contact the client or family to make arrangements for the initial visit. Keep in mind that the client is probably in a weakened condition from recent hospitalization or illness. Let the client know that the initial visit is going to take longer than the remainder of the intermittent visits because of the required paperwork and procedures that accompany the start of care. This initial phone call to the client is a good time to verify directions to the home.

Once you have talked with the client or a family member on the phone, you should have a good indication whether she/he will want to accept the services. Since there are several forms to be filled out during the client's admission, you might want to fill in some of the routine information, such as the client's name and number, on all the forms. This will save time when you are at the client's home. The exception to this practice would be if you receive an indication from the client that she/he is not sure about accepting the services. Organize the paperwork in the the order that you will use it. Most agencies will have admission packets already made up for the staff's use. This saves time when a referral is made. It also helps save you from arriving at the client's home and discovering that a crucial form has been forgotten.

Individual practitioners develop their own routines for the initial visit. Remember, however, that no skilled therapy can be rendered until the service agreement has been signed by the client, since that is his or her indication of giving informed consent for treatment. Occasionally, the individual who is admitting the client is not able to make the initial visit before one of the other agency staff members is scheduled to provide services. For example, the client may require dressing changes twice a day; there may not be a registered nurse (RN) available to change the first dressing and admit the client but a licensed practical or vocational nurse (LPN, LVN) is available. The LPN could take the service agreement when making the visit to change the first dressing. Then the RN can take care of the rest of the paperwork when admitting the client.

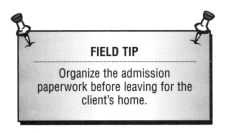

FIELD TIP

Organize the admission paperwork before leaving for the client's home.

ARRIVAL AT CLIENT'S HOME

When you first arrive at a client's home, keep in mind that you are a guest. It is easier to remember that principle when you are in a home than when the client is in a health care facility. You are going to need some room to fill out the forms and organize the paperwork. It is easier to find space in some homes than in others. Be sure that the space you select is with the approval of the family.

Medicare or Insurance Card

You might begin the admission process by asking the client or a family member to get the client's Medicare card or insurance card and all of the medications currently taken by the client. Make a point of specifying both prescription and over-the-counter medications are needed. Don't be surprised if the client brings out a large box full of pill bottles.

If the client is Medicare-eligible, you need to document verification of the Medicare card, the number, and the effective date of eligibility. If the payor is insurance or another type of third-party payor, document the group, individual numbers, and the agency's phone number. Even if the care is covered by Medicare, it is helpful, if the client has secondary insurance, to record that information. If some expenses develop that are not covered by Medicare, such as intravenous (IV) antibiotics, the agency can check with the payor on behalf of the client to inquire if they will pay for the extra expense.

Medications

Record all medications that the client is currently taking. It is helpful if you classify each drug so it is easier to identify drugs with similar actions. You are responsible for verifying that there are no serious drug–drug or drug–food interactions, significant side-effects, or duplication of drugs. The client's pharmacist is a good resource to examine all the drugs for adverse interactions. There are also computer programs that review all of the client's medications and provide potential adverse side-effects, drug reactions, and significant drug–drug and drug–food interactions. Some of these programs also provide teaching handouts about the drugs for the client.

You may find that the client is taking two medications with the same action, which may have been prescribed by two different physicians. You need to verify that the primary physician is aware of the medication duplication. Indicate in the record medications that are new to the client and ones that are changed. These drugs in particular need to be addressed in your teaching plan.

While you are recording the client's medications, you should also record the client's pharmacy and its phone number so it is readily available if you need to phone them in the future. This is a good time to remember to ask the client about any allergies.

As you complete forms, you may want to put them aside in a folder, so you are not reshuffling papers unnecessarily. There are usually several forms that need to be signed by the client on the initial visit. You may want to have the client sign them all at one time. Set those forms aside in a pile until you have them all filled in. You can reassure him or her that this will be the only visit when so many forms need to be signed. Explain each form to the client as she/he signs it.

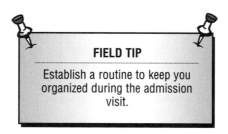

FIELD TIP

Establish a routine to keep you organized during the admission visit.

Home health agencies provide a folder for the client to be left in the home. This folder serves two purposes. First it provides a file for the client's copy of any signed agreements, such as the service agreement and information forms. Second, it is a common file for information used by the agency staff, such as the Certified Nursing Assistant (CNA) care plan. Explain to the client and family the purpose of the folder and ask them to keep it in a place that will be accessible to the staff. It is not wise to leave copies of the client assessment or the visit notes so the client's confidentiality is not jeopardized. Explain each form to the client and family as you add it to the folder. Encourage them to reread the materials later.

Advanced Directives

One informational flyer that is usually contained in the folder is a handout explaining advanced directives. When you are pointing out this pamphlet, it is also a good time to ask if the client has a Living Will and/or a Durable Power of Attorney for Health Care. If so, ask the client to provide a copy for the agency so that the staff can honor the documents. If the client is interested in initiating an advanced directive document but needs assistance, the medical social worker is a good resource for this purpose. Advanced directives cannot be the sole reason for social work services, however. During this discussion, it is also a good time to find out if the client wishes to sign a "Do Not Resuscitate/Intubate" form. Do not assume that a client who has a living will does not want to be resuscitated. Likewise don't assume that a client who does not have a living will does want to be resuscitated.

Client Bill of Rights

Each agency must provide all clients with a written copy and explanation of the Client Bill of Rights and Responsibilities before initiation of treatment. This is usually a one- to two-page document that contains a great deal of information. You could spend 30 to 60 minutes just discussing the bill of rights with the client and family. You can save some time if you let the client and family member read the document while you are filling out some of the paperwork. Encourage them to ask questions about any part that they do not understand. At some point during the visit, review the document and summarize the important points.

An especially crucial aspect of the bill of rights is that the client and family understand who they can call if they are dissatisfied with the care. Names and telephone numbers should be included so the client does not have to seek out this information on his/her own. The agency director and the state authority that handle home care or medical complaints should be listed. Many states require that you have the client sign the bill of rights or its addendum to acknowledge that the document is understood. There must be documentation verifying that the client has received a copy of the rights. Chapter 10, Legal Aspects, contains an in-depth discussion about Advanced Directives, Do Not Rescuscitate orders, and the Client Bill of Rights.

Determination of Primary Payor

Each agency is required to complete a "Determination of the Primary Payor for Medicare Beneficiaries" form with each potential Medicare client during the admission process. The questionnaire explores all other potential payors that may be responsible for payment of the client's care. It is intended that the form be completed with the client's input. The first question asks if the client meets all Medicare home health coverage criteria. If the answer is no, that is all that needs to be completed. If the answer is yes, further questions need to be completed. The form goes on to explore the possibility of other payors such as a hospice, a health maintenance organization (HMO), the Veterans Administration (VA), auto insurance, or medical insurance. This form must be signed by the client to indicate that she/he participated in completing the form and that the information that she/he gave was valid. If the information is found to be invalid, the client agrees to be responsible for payment of the services. Before the client signs the form, make sure that the client understands what the signature implies.

The Medicare regulations state that clients have the right to be advised verbally and in writing of the extent to which payment for home health services may be expected from Medicare. They also need to be informed about what is their financial responsibility. This needs to be reflected on the service agreement. If all or part of the services are not covered by Medicare, the client also needs to sign a form providing a non-coverage notice. If the client fits the profile of an eligible Medicare recipient but does not fit one of the conditions of participation (COP) criteria, such as reasonable and necessary services, or if there is a different primary payor such as an HMO, a non-coverage notice needs to be signed. Another example would be if all the home health services for the client are reimbursable except for an IV antibiotic or a tube feeding; a non-coverage notice needs to be signed in this case. This notice is required to ensure that it is clear to the client and it is documented what will be covered by Medicare and what the client needs to pay for. The form must be signed at any time during care that the agency becomes aware of non-coverage of a service by Medicare. It can be that the services do not meet requirements at the start of care or it may be requirements are met at start of care but that requirements no longer are met later because the client is no longer homebound. It may be that the type of service does not qualify as a skilled service, such as a venipuncture. With this notice, the client has the choice to discontinue services, find another payor, or pay for the services.

SERVICE AGREEMENT

Before completing the service agreement, you need to determine with the help of the client and family which services are needed. For example, do they qualify for and need skilled interventions or do they need home health aide services? Frequently the doctor has already provided orders for all of the needed disciplines, including a home health aide. But it is the client and family who know best if the nursing assistant is really needed. The doctor expects that the case manager will assess the client needs. Be sure that the client and family members understand that once the skilled services are no longer needed, the aide services will be discontinued. It helps to remind the client about this regulation from time to time throughout the client's care. Clients seem to feel more lost without the certified nursing assistant (CNA) services than any of the other disciplines.

Once Medicare eligibility has been determined and the assessment determines a need for skilled and unskilled services, the service agreement can be completed. Each agency will vary the format of the service agreement but there are basic requirements that all agencies follow. There will be a statement that indicates the client consents to receiving treatment from the agency staff. The form will indicate what services are available through the agency.

An important section is the one that includes the specific services that will be provided, the payor for the services, and the client's financial responsibility. This section needs to be filled in completely before the client signs the agreement. If any changes are made later, a new agreement needs to be signed by the client. The original agreement is retained in the client record along with the new agreeement.

Frequency and Duration

Determining the need for the specific types of services is usually the easy part. It's specifying the frequency and duration of those services that poses the challenge, especially for the practitioner who is new to home care. Usually the skilled services have already been determined by the physician. Sometimes the doctor has also specified the frequency and duration of the services but in most cases, the physician expects that home care professionals will use their expertise to determine those factors.

The frequency of visits are the number of visits that practitioners of a particular discipline will make per week to treat the client. The duration is the number of weeks that the services at the specified frequency will be provided. Short ranges are allowed to be used, but their regular use is not recommended. (Short ranges are a variance of one day such as 1 to 2 days per week.) A range of no more than two visits per week will be accepted.

A week can be based upon the agency's work week or a client week. For some agencies the week begins on Sunday and ends on Saturday, whereas for others it begins on Monday and ends on Sunday. A client week would begin on the first day of the start of care. The system used should be consistent within the agency.

The following provides an example for writing a frequency and duration statement. Your agency uses a Sunday to Saturday week and you determine that the client requires three visits of skilled nursing or therapy per week (Monday-Wednesday-Friday) for 5 weeks. You admit the client on a Wednesday. Therefore you will be seeing the client twice that week, on Wednesday and Friday. The documentation of the frequency and duration for this situation can be stated in the following way:

SN services: 2 × 1wk; 3 × 4 wks.

If you are including another professional discipline on the service agreement, you are not in a position to determine that discipline's frequency and duration but you do know that an evaluation needs to be made. Therefore document it as:

PT services: Eval, Frequency and Duration to follow.

Following are some suggested frequencies. Keep in mind that all clients are individuals and some will require less frequent visits and others more frequent visits than the suggested numbers. These frequencies are intended to be used as guidelines only.

Post-hospitalization:	3 to 5 times per week for 2 weeks
	2 to 3 times per week for 1 week
	1 to 2 times per week for 1 week
Medical condition (stable):	3 to 4 times per week for 1 week
	2 to 4 times per week for 2 weeks
Medical condition (unstable):	5 to 7 times per week for 1 week
	3 to 5 times per week for 3 weeks
	1 to 3 times per week for 4 weeks

As Needed (PRN) Visits

Frequency ranges are not meant to be used for a situation in which a client needs assistance outside the scheduled times. For example, a client with a Foley catheter who discovers in the evening that the catheter is plugged, cannot wait for the next regularly scheduled visit to have the catheter changed. This situation is a reasonable expectation for a client with a catheter, so the admitting nurse should anticipate the need for as needed (PRN) visits.

The number of PRN visits per certification period needs to be limited. Each fiscal intermediary may interpret this regulation differently. Home care professionals must be informed about the number of PRN visits allowed by their agency's fiscal intermediary. If more than the allowed number of PRN visits are provided within the certification period, those visits will be reviewed by the fiscal intermediary to determine if the visits were medically necessary; there is not an automatic denial of payment after the allowed number of visits.

Another type of client that you could anticipate would need PRN visits is a client with an intravenous line. When indicating the need for PRN visits, make sure you provide justification for that extra visit. If an extra visit is needed for a client without a PRN order, a verbal physician's order must be obtained before the nurse makes the visit.

Frequency and Duration for Home Health Aide Visits

The frequency and duration of visits for the home health aide (HHA) needs to be specific; no ranges are allowed. Usually, the frequencies for HHA visits are three to five visits per week. Medicare will pay for daily visits, as long as they are justified. Usually such frequent visits are justified if the client is bedbound and incontinent or has a draining wound. Of course, this is expected to be a temporary situation. Documentation needs to indicate that the client and family caregiver are either not willing or able to provide the personal care.

It is expected that the frequencies and durations will be followed as specified for all disciplines. The visits each week should not be less or more than the number ordered. If there is a discrepancy in the number of visits for a given week, a doctor's order is needed to cover it.

Payor

The payor needs to be specified for each service provided for the client. Sometimes there may be two or three payors for a given client. Medicare may be paying for skilled nursing, therapy, and a CNA. Insurance may be paying for the tube feeding. Medicaid may be paying for some respite care for the client's caregiver.

Client Financial Responsibility

The client financial responsibility part of the form is a crucial section that needs to be accurately completed. Federal and state governments are especially strict regarding this section. It is crucial that the clients and their families know what they are expected to pay, if anything, for the services.

If Medicare is the payor for all of the services and, as in most cases, the client is not responsible for any payment, you need to write none or 0 in this section for each service. If the client is responsible for part of the service, such as the IV drugs, that needs to be specified, including the amount the client should expect to pay either per dose, per day, or per week. If the agency has an individual, such as an admission nurse, who is responsible for all of the referrals that come in; that person will probably obtain and record the exact amounts for you. But if you are expected to obtain that information, you will need to phone the pharmacy or durable medical equipment company who will be providing the supplies to find out the client's cost.

If the payor is an HMO, preferred provider organization (PPO), or another kind of insurance, there may be a deductible or co-payment that the client needs to pay. There also may be a policy limit or benefit limit (cap) for the coverage. Those amounts should all be included on the agreement.

Special Authorizations

The service agreement includes an authorization from the client for the agency to bill and receive payment from the appropriate payor. Most agreements will provide written expectations in case of agreement termination by the client or if the client privately hires one of the agency's employees. Another important statement to be included in this document is an authorization to release information from the doctor, facility in which the client had been a patient, or any other source that has relevant information for the client's care. This authorization includes an agreement giving permission for the agency to release information to the third-party payors and other health care providers involved in the care of the client.

Most service agreements include a section for the client to indicate whether they have prepared an advanced directive. If there is an indication of a living will or medical power of attorney, or both, the nurse or therapist needs to record that a copy of this document was obtained or that the client was instructed to provide a copy for the agency. This section might be a good place to record this statement if there is enough space. Most agencies try to include all of the basic information that needs to be signed by the client in this one document so the client does not have to sign several documents. The home health professional needs to review all of the sections in the agreement with the client before it is signed to be sure the client understands everything in the document.

Signature Page

The signature page needs to allow for all of the possible scenarios. In other words, there needs to be a place for the client to sign or for someone else to sign if the client cannot do so. Keep in mind that if someone else signs the form for the client, that person needs to have a legal power of attorney to do so.

If the client does not speak English, it is ideal to have the service agreement written in the client's language. There needs to be documentation to indicate that there was a translator present and who that person was. If the nurse or therapist happens to be bilingual and able to communicate fluently with the client, it would be wise to indicate that on the signature page. This helps a surveyor understand that the client was well informed about the document that was being signed.

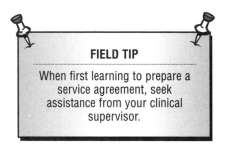

FIELD TIP

When first learning to prepare a service agreement, seek assistance from your clinical supervisor.

Care Plan for Home Health Aide

If HHA services are to be provided, a care plan needs to be written for the nursing assistant to follow. State law may designate who can develop that plan. Some states may indicate that only a registered nurse can develop the HHA plan, whereas other states may allow either a RN or a therapist to develop and supervise the care plan. Chapter 8, Case Manager Responsibilities, discusses the HHA care plan in more detail.

A copy of the care plan needs to be left in the home so it is available to any CNA who cares for the client. This requirement can pose a dilemma for the individual who is admitting the client. The admission process does take extra time and can be tiring for the client, so the person processing the admission would not want to spend any unnecessary time in the home. If the first aide visit is not scheduled for a day or so, you could make out the care plan later at the office and then send the copy with the CNA who makes the first visit. This nursing assistant will be instructed to place it in the client's home folder. If the first HHA visit is scheduled for the same day as the admission visit, the nurse or therapist will need to make out the plan during the admission visit. It helps the client if there is an information sheet that explains the role of the nursing assistant and what duties that individual can provide during the visit. This form can be left in the client's folder for the client and family to read at their leisure

HOME SAFETY ASSESSMENT

Chapter 13, Safety Issues provides a detailed discussion about the safety assessment of the client's home and about classifying the client's priority in case of a disaster. It is expected that these assessments are made and documented during the admission visit. This does not mean that this visit is the only time to assess for safety. Such evaluation should be done on an on-going basis. Basically, the home situation is assessed for features to prevent falls and provide fire and electrical safety, medication use safety, and an emergency preparedness plan.

The emergency preparedness plan needs to focus on the evacuation plan for the client from the home in case of a fire or another emergency. Additionally, it needs to include alternate care arrangements for the client in case of a disaster. For example, where would the client go if the home became flooded or lost its electricity? It may be to a friend's or a relative's home or it may have to be a temporary shelter. It is helpful to have these questions answered before there actually is an emergency or disaster situation.

CLIENT ASSESSMENT

Once the client has signed the service agreement, you can begin the client assessment and treatment. This initial assessment involves a thorough review of all the body systems. Also integrated throughout the assessment process are the OASIS items that need to be transmitted to the Health Care Financing Administration (HCFA). Appendix A provides a guide for the History and Systems Review.

The initial assessment for the home health client tends to be more comprehensive than that performed when a client is admitted to a structured facility. This is because there are usually other professionals contributing to the assessment data in the structured facility. The assessment begins with the basic demographic information about the client. When recording information about the client's diagnoses, obtain accurate dates of onset and exacerbation. If the exacerbation dates are not recorded, it may give the impression that the client's condition is chronic and does not justify Medicare reimbursement.

Routine vital signs are taken. Two different blood pressure measurements should be taken during the initial assessment. Preferably, one should be taken with the client in the sitting position and one with the client standing so orthostatic hypotension can be detected. Of course, your ability to make these measurements depends on the client's ability to sit and stand. If the client is bedbound, obtain a blood pressure reading from each arm.

The psychosocial assessment needs to answer the following questions: Is there a primary caregiver for the client? Is the caregiver readily available to the client? What is the client's understanding of the disease? Does the client live alone? Is the caregiver willing, able, and available? Does the client or caregiver have the capacity to learn new material?

OASIS

OASIS or the Outcome and Assessment Information Set is a group of data elements that all Medicare-certified home health agencies are required by HCFA to gather. Additional OASIS information can be found in Chapter 3, Conditions of Participation. The data items do not constitute a comprehensive assessment; therefore, each agency needs to complete the tool with the assessment items that are missing. Each OASIS item has an identifier that consists of five characters: one letter, which is an M, and four numbers, the first number being zero. Since the first two characters are M0, you will often hear them referred to as M0 items. All M0 items must be completed at the designated times, including at the start of care.

These items must be answered as written; they cannot be altered. However, the items do not have to be asked in the same sequence as they are numbered. They can be integrated into the agency assessment tool in any way, as long as they are left intact and none are eliminated. Some items can be determined when calling the client to set up the appointment for the initial assessment. These items are M0770, assess ability to use telephone; M0400, hearing and auditory comprehension of language; M0410, speech and oral expression of language; and M0560, cognitive functioning. Table 6–1 provides some examples of the OASIS items. Notice that most of the examples do not give you the option of checking a box to indicate the item does not apply. It forces you to choose one of the other answers. You do not have the option to add not applicable (NA). The intent is that the use of selections Not Applicable and Unknown, even when offered, be kept to a minimum. The Unknown selection usually implies that more information about the client needs to be obtained.

The response that is chosen for each item should be the one that best describes the client's status most of the time during the day of the assessment. Some items inquire about events occurring within the past 14 days or at a specific point of time. These items need to be followed exactly. Collection of the data will involve direct observation, interviews, or a combination of both interview and observation. The direct observation is preferred but not always practical. When using interview data, the client should be the primary source of information.

All items must be answered, except when one item instructs you to skip some other. If the tool being used is integrated with assessment items in addition to the OASIS items, be sure you only skip the M0 items. Usually there is only one answer for each M0 item, except for a few that instruct you to "Mark all that apply."

You can write comments about the client next to the item to clarify your selection. The extra comments will not be transmitted as data. As discussed in the chapter on documentation, you need to provide wound measurements in centimeters. If the assessment tool does not have a special section for that information, it could be written next to the M0 item(s) concerning the client's wound.

If you are new to home health, it may be an advantage that all of the paperwork is new to you. Presently all home health personnel are adjusting to new paperwork. Whether you are new to home health or just new to OASIS, the amount of OASIS paperwork can be intimidating. The OASIS pilot studies have shown that completing the documents consumes more time at first, but as home health professionals become accustomed to the items, they are able to complete the paperwork in the same amount of time or less as they did the previous paperwork. Although there are several pages to the assessment tool, the check box format facilitates efficient recording.

When first using the OASIS items, you may need guidance from your supervisor to answer each item accurately. Not only is accuracy important for the client's care but it is also crucial for accurate data to be transmitted to HCFA. These data will be used to help determine reimbursement amounts for the agency and region, once the prospective payment system is implemented.

The OASIS items concerning wounds do not deal with all types of wounds, so do not try to fit a wound into an item if it just does not fit. The OASIS wound items deal with pressure ulcers (resulting from tissue hypoxia due to prolonged pressure), stasis ulcers (due to inadequate venous circulation), and surgical wounds. Included under surgical wounds are central line sites, orthopedic pin sites, stapled or sutured incisions, drain sites, debrided graft sites, and mediport sites. Scars or keloid formations from prior surgical wounds are not considered surgical wounds as far as OASIS data are concerned. If a wound has more than one opening, consider each opening as a

Table 6–1	OASIS ITEM EXAMPLES

(M0300) CURRENT RESIDENCE:

1 – Patient's owned or rented residence (house, apartment, or mobile home owned or rented by patient/couple/significant other)
2 – Family member's residence
3 – Boarding home or rented room
4 – Board and care or assisted living facility
5 – Other (specify) _____

(M0680) TOILETING: ABILITY TO GET TO AND FROM THE TOILET OR BEDSIDE COMMODE.

Prior Current

0 – Able to get to and from the toilet independently with or without a device.
1 – When reminded, assisted, or supervised by another person, able to get to and from the toilet.
2 – *Unable* to get to and from the toilet but is able to use a bedside commode (with or without assistance).
3 – *Unable* to get to and from the toilet or bedside commode but is able to use a bedpan/urinal independently.
4 – Is totally dependent in toileting.
   UK – Unknown
If score is not 0 – Able, willing, and capable caregiver name _____

(M0700) AMBULATION/LOCOMOTION: ABILITY TO *SAFELY* WALK, ONCE IN A STANDING POSITION, OR USE A WHEELCHAIR, ONCE IN A SEATED POSITION, ON A VARIETY OF SURFACES.

Prior Current

0 – Able to independently walk on even and uneven surfaces and climb stairs with or without railings (i.e., needs no human assistance or assistive device).
1 – Requires use of a device (e.g., cane, walker) to walk alone *or* requires human supervision or assistance to negotiate stairs or steps or uneven surfaces.
2 – Able to walk only with the supervision/assistance of another person at all times.
3 – Chair fast, *unable* to ambulate but is able to wheel self.
4 – Chair fast, unable to ambulate and is *unable* to wheel self.
5 – Bedfast, unable to ambulate or be up in a chair.
   UK – Unknown

(M0420) FREQUENCY OF PAIN INTERFERING WITH PATIENT'S ACTIVITY OR MOVEMENT:

0 – Patient has no pain or pain does not interfere with activity or movement.

Table continued on opposite page

| **Table 6–1** | **OASIS ITEM EXAMPLES** *Continued* |

1 – Less often than daily.
2 – Daily, but not constantly.
3 – All of the time.

(M0780) MANAGEMENT OF ORAL MEDICATIONS: *PATIENT'S ABILITY* TO PREPARE AND TAKE ALL PRESCRIBED ORAL MEDICATIONS RELIABLY AND SAFELY, INCLUDING ADMINISTRATION OF THE CORRECT DOSAGE AT THE APPROPRIATE TIMES/INTERVALS. *EXCLUDES* INJECTABLE AND INTRAVENOUS MEDICATIONS. (NOTE: THIS REFERS TO ABILITY, NOT COMPLIANCE OR WILLINGNESS.)

0 – Able to independently take the correct oral medication(s) and proper dosage(s) at the correct times.
1 – Able to take medications(s) at the correct times if:
    (a) individual dosages are prepared in advance by another person; *OR*
    (b) given daily reminders; *OR*
    (c) someone develops a drug diary or chart.
2 – *Unable* to take medication unless administered by someone else.
    NA – No oral medications prescribed.
    UK – Unknown

Adapted from OASIS survey form; version B1 developed by the Center for Health Services and Policy Research, Denver.

separate wound. Burns, ostomies, and gunshot wounds do not fit into any of these three categories. They need to be addressed in another section of the assessment tool as determined by the agency.

Make sure that your answers are consistent. For example, item M0445 asks if the patient has a pressure ulcer. If the answer is no, the item directs the assessor to go to item M0468, but some nurses and therapists still try to complete item M0450, which calls for the staging of a pressure ulcer. This situation makes the reader wonder whether the client does or does not have a pressure ulcer. If the client does have a pressure ulcer(s), be sure to identify all pressure areas including those that are stage 1. If you read the directions written for each OASIS item, you should be able to record accurate information.

OASIS Situations

This section of the chapter contains some client situations. Read them carefully and then choose the correct answer in the OASIS items that follow. The correct answers can be found in Table 6–2.

Situation 1:

Walter Jones, 67 years old, lives with his wife, daughter, and two dogs in a mobile home. He was discharged yesterday from the hospital following abdominal surgery. He is receiving IV antibiotics through a central line at home. Has a 15-cm stapled wound with a Penrose drain in place through a separate incision. Home health aide visits have been arranged for three times a week. When you phoned to make arrangements for the first visit, the client answered the phone and gave you directions to the home.

(M0340) Patient Lives With: (Mark all that apply.)

☐ 1 – Lives alone

☐ 2 – With spouse or significant other

☐ 3 – With other family member

☐ 4 – With a friend

☐ 5 – With paid help (other than home care agency staff)

☐ 6 – With other than above

(M0340) Cognitive Functioning: (Patient's current level of alertness, orientation, comprehension, concentration, and immediate memory for simple commands.)

☐ 0 – Alert/oriented, able to focus and shift attention, comprehends and recalls task directions independently.

☐ 1 – Requires prompting (cuing, repetition, reminders) only under stressful or unfamiliar conditions.

☐ 2 – Requires assistance and some direction in specific situations (e.g., on all tasks involving shifting of attention), or consistently requires low stimulus environment due to distractibility.

❒ 3 – Requires considerable assistance in routine situations. Is not alert and oriented or is unable to shift attention and recall directions more than half the time.

❒ 4 – Totally dependent due to disturbances such as constant disorientation, coma, persistent vegetative state, or delirium.

(M0440) Does this patient have a Skin Lesion or an Open Wound? This excludes "OSTOMIES"

❒ 0 – No (If No, go to M0490)

❒ 1 – Yes

(M0445) Does this patient have a Pressure Ulcer?

❒ 0 – No (If No, go to M0468)

❒ 1 – Yes

(M0468) Does this patient have a Stasis Ulcer?

❒ 0 – No (If No, go to M0482)

❒ 1 – Yes

(M0482) Does this patient have a Surgical Wound?

❒ 0 – No (If No, go to M0490) (skip the remainder of the category)

❒ 1 – Yes

Situation 2:

Patricia Watson, 72 years old, lives with her spouse of 20 years in their home (a three-bedroom house). She was diagnosed with congestive heart failure (CHF) one year ago. She requires 2 liters oxygen continuously. She is able to ambulate short distances (10 feet) before she becomes dyspneic. Most of the time she uses a wheelchair, which she is able to propel. She requires some assistance from her husband for dressing. Sometimes she is forgetful, and her husband needs to remind her to take her oral and inhalant medications.

(M0650) Ability to Dress *Upper* Body (with or without dressing aids) including undergarments, pullovers, front-opening shirts and blouses, managing zippers, buttons, and snaps:

❐ 0 – Able to get clothes out of closets and drawers, put them on and remove them from the upper body without assistance.

❐ 1 – Able to dress upper body without assistance if clothing is laid out or handed to the patient.

❐ 2 – Someone must help the patient put on upper body clothing.

❐ 3 – Patient depends entirely upon another person to dress the upper body. UK-Unknown

If score is not 0–Able, willing and capable caregiver name

_____

(M0490) When is the patient dyspneic or noticeably short of breath?

❐ 0 – Never, patient is not short of breath

❐ 1 – When walking more than 20 feet, climbing stairs

❐ 2 – With moderate exertion (e.g., while dressing, using commode or bedpan, walking distances less than 20 feet)

❐ 3 – With minimal exertion (e.g., while eating, talking, or performing other ADLs) or with agitation

❐ 4 – At rest (during day or night)

(M0790) Management of Inhalant/Mist Medications: *Patient's ability* to prepare and take *all* prescribed inhalant/mist medications (nebulizers, metered dose devices) reliably and safely, including administration of the correct dosage at the appropriate times/intervals. *Excludes* all other forms of medication (oral tablets, injectable, and IV medications).

❐ 0 – Able to independently take the correct medication and proper dosage at the correct times.

❏ 1 – Able to take medication at the correct times if individual dosages are prepared in advance by another
person, *or* given daily reminders.

❏ 2 – *Unable* to take medication unless administered by
someone else.

NA-No inhalant/mist medications prescribed.

UK-Unknown

| Table 6–2 | ANSWERS TO OASIS SITUATIONS |

SITUATION #1: WALTER JONES
(M0340) Patient lives:
2 – With *spouse* or significant other
3 – With other family member (daughter)
(M0560) Cognitive functioning
0 – Alert/oriented (gave directions to home)
(M0440)
1 – Yes, has an open wound
(M0445)
0 – No pressure ulcer
(M0468)
0 – No stasis ulcer
(M0482)
1 – Yes, a surgical wound

SITUATION #2: PATRICIA WATSON
2 – Someone must help patient put on upper body clothing.
(M0490)
2 – With moderate exertion (walking distances less than 20 feet)
(M0790)
1 – Able to take medication at the correct times if:
1 – (b) given daily reminders

SKILLED INTERVENTIONS PERFORMED DURING VISIT

Keep in mind if you do not find a need for at least one skilled intervention during this visit, it is questionable whether skilled services are needed at a later time. Frequently, the problem is more the lack of documentation of the skilled interventions provided rather than the lack of interventions. Be sure to include the reason the client is homebound if it is not already documented. There is always the need for skilled observations and skilled teaching even if there are no particular procedures, such as a dressing change, to be performed. This part of the documentation does not need to be done during the actual visit but can be done when the nurse or therapist returns to the office. By this time the client and family caregiver are probably very tired and need some time to rest. Be sure to make some notes of the collected data so you do not forget them later.

There is usually some need for narrative charting. It is easy to remember to document procedures like IVs started, gait training, and dressing changes, but observations and some teaching are so routine that we frequently forget to record them. Some items that should be included, if there is no other designated area for them, are documentation that the client was informed about the Bill of Rights, Advanced Directives including disposition of copies of the documents, community resources, and the discharge plan. Any skilled teaching about the client's condition, safety measures, use of DME, and medication precautions also needs to be documented. Additionally, any skilled observations, such as cardiopulmonary or integumentary systems, need to be specified. The narrative summary should include all of the needs and concerns identified in the assessment that apply to the skilled care that will be provided.

PLAN OF CARE

Once the client assessment has been completed, the problem list can be formulated. First you should re-examine the client's diagnoses to prioritize them in terms of their relation to the client's need for skilled interventions. The primary diagnosis should reflect the reason the skilled care is being provided.

Example #1. The client may have diagnoses of chronic congestive heart failure and diabetes mellitus but home care was ordered because the client requires wound care for an ulcer on the foot. The primary diagnosis should be diabetes with ulcer manifestation.

Example #2. A client with an old cerebrovascular accident (CVA) requires physical therapy following hip replacement for a fractured hip. The primary diagnosis should be Joint Replacement.

Example #3. A client with a recent CVA requires speech language therapy for dysphagia. The primary diagnosis should be Dysphagia.

If there is need for practitioners from more than one discipline to provide skilled interventions, there needs to be a diagnosis that justifies each skill. For example, nursing may be needed for wound care for the client with diabetes but physical therapy is also needed because the client had a recent fractured fibula. The primary diagnosis is the condition for which the greatest amount of care is being rendered. The secondary diagnoses are additional diagnoses being treated. Most likely, diabetes with ulcer manifestation would be the primary diagnosis and fractured fibula would be a secondary diagnosis.

ICD-9-CM Codes

Some agencies require the field staff to designate the ICD-9-CM codes for the client diagnoses. ICD-9-CM stands for the International Classification of Diseases-Ninth Edition-Clinical Modification. Other agencies have the ICD-9-CM codes entered by data entry clerks. If you work for the former type of agency, each agency has a list of the codes, which are updated on a yearly basis. If you work for the second type of agency, you still must record the diagnoses accurately so the data entry personnel know which code is appropriate for the given diagnoses. This means that you need to be familiar with how the diagnoses are stated. Along with the ICD-9-CM codes, make sure that you have verified the most current dates of onset or exacerbation for each diagnosis.

Client Problems

As in the nursing process, the next step in the plan of care is to identify the client problems. The North American Nursing Diagnosis Association (NANDA) Approved Nursing Diagnoses meets this need. Table 6–3 provides diagnoses used most frequently for the home health client. The etiology of each condition should be reflected in the client assessment. If there is not evidence of that cause found during assessment, it is either because the etiology is not appropriate for the client's condition or the assessment is incomplete.

When selecting the appropriate diagnoses for the client, do not overdo it. Some clients could have several problems that you may be tempted to solve, but you have to be reasonable. Any problems that you identify need to be addressed on a regular basis throughout the client's care or until they are resolved. You have a limited period of time to care for the client and some of these may be long-term problems.

Table 6–3	HOME HEALTH CLIENT DIAGNOSES

Knowledge deficit
Potential for/self-care deficit
Potential for/impaired mobility
Potential for/altered nutrition
Potential for/presence of injury
Potential for/altered comfort/pain
Potential for/altered health maintenance
Potential for/impaired home maintenance
Potential for/impaired skin integrity
Potential for/altered thought process
Potential for/altered elimination
Potential for/altered cardiac status
Potential for/ineffective breathing/airway
Potential for/impaired social interaction
Potential for/altered sensory/perceptual
Potential for/presence of infection
Potential for/ineffective coping
Potential for/altered growth/development
Potential for/anticipatory grieving

You may identify some client problems that are already being managed by the client and family. For example, the client with chronic obstructive pulmonary disease may have episodes of pneumonia, but your initial assessment reveals that she/he knows how to observe for early signs of complications and when to see the doctor for treatment. You need to focus on the problems related to the client's current diagnoses. It would not be appropriate to treat a client for a problem that is already being managed effectively.

The plan of care needs to specify the frequency and duration of services. Granted you have already specified the frequency and duration on the service agreement but it also needs to be specified here. This information is recorded on the HCFA 485 form, which eventually is sent to the physician as the client's orders for his/her signature. Frequencies and durations need to be accurate. If either the frequency or duration is altered, a new doctor's order needs to be obtained.

Skilled Interventions

Once you have identified the client's problems, you need to specify the skilled interventions required to manage those problems. There are three major categories of interventions to be considered: skilled observations, teaching, and administration. The observations may include cardiovascular, integumentary, musculoskeletal, or any of the other body systems depending on what is appropriate for the client's diagnoses. If you include vital signs, specify the parameters that each sign should fall within. These parameters become part of the doctor's orders.

Skilled teaching must address any learning needs of the client and the caregiver(s). If there is an indication that the client is receiving any new or changed medications, there needs to be teaching in relation to those medications. You may need to teach the client and family member(s) how to perform a specific procedure such as a dressing change, insulin administration, or tracheostomy care. If the client and family do not understand the disease process of the client's condition, that teaching needs to be included in the plan of care. If the client has a terminal condition, the client and family need to learn about what to expect as the client's condition progresses. Find an opportunity to educate the client and family about their responsibilities as recipients of home health care. Many agencies have checklists of all the common skilled interventions that help provide cues for the staff members so important ones are not forgotten.

The skilled administration of treatments is frequently specified in the initial doctor's orders. You may, however, discover other treatment needs that the doctor has not thought of that should be included. It can take up to 20 to 30 days to process the Plan of Care and receive the signed orders from the physician; therefore, you need to obtain verbal orders to cover any additional treatments while you are waiting for the return of the signed plan. The interventions need to include any home health aide services that are needed.

Client Goals

Client goals need to be included in the plan of care. The goals need to relate to the client's problems and the interventions intended. Make sure they are reasonable goals to be accomplished by your discipline before the specified end date. The goals and end dates could have already been determined by the primary payor if that payor is not Medicare. Keep in mind that you need to address each goal on a regular basis. The outcome date needs to be specified, so there is sufficient time for the client to reach the goal but not so long that the client care continues indefinitely. The HCFA staff expects that some clients' care will need to continue beyond the certification period (no longer than 62 days) but they do expect that the goals will be achieved in a timely manner. They also expect that any client care that extends beyond the certification period is justified in the documentation. If the goal is not achieved by the outcome date, the record needs to reflect why the goal needs to be extended. Goals need to include those for the home health aide. Table 6–4 provides a list of suggested goals that are appropriate for home health clients.

Table 6–4	SUGGESTED CLIENT GOALS

Wound (specify location) healed without complications.
Pain will be controlled with use of prescribed analgesic.
Patient/caregiver will demonstrate correct procedure for dressing change.
No evidence of complications of diabetes.
Patient will be independent in activities of daily living.
Patient/caregiver will indicate knowledge regarding disease process.
Patient will indicate knowledge of medications.
Patient independent in ambulation with walker.
Patient/caregiver able to demonstrate correct insulin
    preparation and administration.

Discharge Plans

Discharge plans should be identified at the start of care. The sooner the client and family become aware of the discharge plan and the goals to be achieved before discharge, the sooner everyone is going to be able to work together to achieve reasonable goals. It helps the clients who think that services should be forever and those who prefer that services be limited to develop reasonable expectations for the length of home care.

HCFA-485

The Home Health Certification and Plan of Care is a form provided by HCFA to record the client's plan of care and be signed by the doctor. This form is commonly referred to as the HFCA-485 or simply as 485, which is the form number. A copy of this form can be found in Appendix B.

Most agencies have a data entry clerk to transfer the information from the initial visit documentation to the 485, but you may be working for an agency that requires the field staff to complete the 485. Even if you are not required to actually complete the form, your documentation needs to be clear and accurate so the data entry clerk does not have to guess about the information that needs to be entered. Once this form is signed by the doctor, a copy of it is placed in the client record and is available if the fiscal intermediary requests a copy be sent to them.

All 28 fields of the 485 form must be completed. The data for most of the fields have already been gathered using the OASIS items. The top of the form calls for the client's demographic data including client number and start of care date (SOC). It also contains the dates of the certification period. The first date of the certification period is the start of care date (first day client seen by agency staff). The last day of the certification period is two months from the SOC date. For example, if the SOC date is February 20, 2000, then the Certification dates would be 02/20/00 to 04/20/00. The number of days varies according to the number of days in the particular months involved (58–62 days). The last day of the certification period becomes the first day of the next period if the client's case is recertified.

The 485 form must contain all pertinent diagnoses and either the onset dates or the date of the most recent exacerbation. All medications being taken by the client, including over-the-counter products and respiratory inhalants, their dose, frequency, route of administration, and whether they are new or changed are recorded on the form. DME, supplies, safety measures, nutritional requirements, and allergies are included. If the DME and supplies field is incomplete, it may result in non-coverage of supplies. There is a checklist on which to indicate the client's functional limitations, activities permitted, mental status, and prognosis. If functional limitations are not documented, Medicare may deny payment for services provided. An indication of a decreased activity level may imply the need to refer the client for physical or occupational therapy services. When completing the prognosis section, keep in mind what your response implies. If the response is excellent, the implication is that the client will need just short-term home care.

The order section specifies each skilled and unskilled discipline and treatments done by each. Each discipline will specify the amount, frequency, and duration of service. Next is listed the client's goals, rehabilitation potential, and discharge plans. The responses given to the OASIS items provide guidelines for the discharge plans.

The lower section of the 485 contains areas for the nurse's signature and date of verbal SOC. In other words, the nurse who obtains the original verbal orders from the doctor signs the form and records the date that the verbal orders were obtained. The physician's name and address follow. Last, is a section for the physician's signature and date signed. The signature approves the plan of care and certifies that the patient is homebound and requires skilled care. Frequently, the orders are returned to the agency, signed by the doctor but without a date of the signature. HCFA will accept a form that was not dated by the physician as long as the agency stamps the date on the form when it is returned to the office. If the form does not contain any date, HCFA will consider any visits covered by those orders invalid.

Verbal orders are needed to cover services from the SOC date until the physician signs the plan of care. That verbal order must be documented in the medical record. The plan of care or verbal orders may be transmitted by facsimile machine. Some physicians prefer to use the fax machine and others don't. It is helpful if the agency maintains an updated book or file of physician preferences and any signed standing orders. Written authorizations need to be obtained from any non-Medicare payors involved in the case. More and more third-party payors will not pay for services unless they have provided prior written authorizations.

The signed plan of care needs to be returned to the agency office as soon as practical after the start of care date. Some states may specify a particular time period. The expected time is usually 30 days. Most agencies try to have orders signed and returned within 20 days. You may say that sounds like a lot of time, but if you look at the flow of paperwork in your office, you will see how a short delay of handling the client's chart, anywhere along the way, can throw the time line off. All offices handle the paper flow differently but the following diagram will help provide for you an idea of the admission process.

It is crucial that the admission paperwork is completed and returned to the office within the scheduled timeframe. If the paperwork is due within 48 hours from the SOC but is not returned until 5 days following the SOC, you can see how that delay pushes back the time line and can mean that the orders are not returned until much later than the 30-day requirement.

Another factor is that OASIS data are required to be entered for transmission within 7 days of the SOC. The payor cannot be billed for any services relating to that client's care until the signed orders are back in the office. It is possible that the agency might not receive reimbursement for some visits because of late orders. That delay can also affect the time when not only the admitting case manager receives payment for the visit but any other discipline that is providing treatment.

ADMISSION PAPER FLOW
REFERRAL
↓
ADMISSION PAPERWORK INITIATED
↓
RN/THERAPIST ASSIGNED TO CASE
↓
CLIENT ADMITTED TO SERVICES
↓
COMPLETED ADMISSION PACKET RETURNED TO OFFICE
↓
CLIENT CHART ASSEMBLED
↓
CHART GOES TO AUDITOR (CHECKED FOR COMPLETENESS)
↓
DATA ENTRY (485 CREATED + PAYROLL DATA ENTRY)
↓
SCHEDULES CREATED FOR RN/THERAPIST/AIDE
↓
CLINICAL SUPERVISOR (COMPLETE AUDIT OF CHART)
↓
CHART TO RECORDS DEPARTMENT
↓
ORDERS SENT TO PHYSICIAN

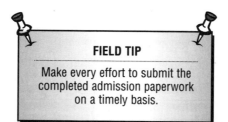

FIELD TIP

Make every effort to submit the completed admission paperwork on a timely basis.

References

A Homecare Therapist Guide to Medicare Service Delivery. The Beacon Homecare FOCUS Series. Medicare Reimbursement for Therapy Services, pp. 1–9, Mequon, WI, Beacon Health, 1996.

Crisler, K. S.: Oasis: What it is and How to Implement and Integrate it in a Home Care Agency, pp. 1–11. Denver, Center for Health Services and Policy Research, 1998.

Health Care Financing Administration: Home Health Agency Manual (HIM-11), Coverage of Services, Sec. 200, pp. 11–24 Washington, D.C., Department of Health and Human Services 1987.

Health Care Financing Administration: Home Health Agency Manual (HIM-11), Entitlement Verification Procedures, Sec. 340, pp. 32–32.4 Washington, D.C., Department of Health and Human Services. 1992.

Health Care Financing Administration: Home Health Agency Manual (HIM-11), Coverage of Services, Sec. 234, pp. 11–24. Washington, D.C., Department of Health and Human Services. 1998.

Health Care Financing Administration: OASIS Implementation Manual, Attachment A: General OASIS Instructions, pp. 8.11–8.12 Attachment B, pp. 8.26–8.75. Washington, D.C., Department of Health and Human Services. 1998.

Hilliard, L. S.: Manager's Corner: Innovative or Disintegrate. Home Care Nurse News, 1998; 5(6):1–2, 8.

Hogue, E.: The Behavioral Offset of the Interim Payment System: What HCFA Expects Home Care Providers to do. Arizona Homefront, 1998; 15(6):10–11.

Hospital and Payor ICD-9-CM, Vol 1,2,3. Salt Lake City, Medicode Inc., 1998.

Management and Evaluation of a Care Plan. The Beacon Homecare FOCUS Series, pp. 1–16. Mequon, WI, Beacon Health, 1996.

Medicare Bulletin #415, by bcc (Blue Cross Calif) Fiscal Intermediary, Oxnard, CA, May 4, 1998.

Medicare Bulletin #416, by bcc (Blue Cross Calif) Fiscal Intermediary, Oxnard, CA, July 13, 1998, p. 13.

Medicare Reimbursement of Therapy Services. The Beacon Homecare FOCUS Series, 1996; pp. 1–9.

Olsten Health Services: Continuing Nurses Education, pp. 12–5 to 12–15. Melville, NY, Olsten Health Services, 1996.

Olsten Health Services: Training and Development, OHM/Introduction to Medicare SSG, 1/97. pp. 1–3 to 1–17, 3–3 to 3–4, 4–3 to 4–6. Melville, NY, Olsten Health Services, 1997.

Olsten Health Services: Training and Development, Aide-level training program, Module 1, 1/97. pp. 1–9 to 1–12. Melville, NY, Olsten Health Services, 1997.

Polzien, G., Kendall, B., and Hindelang, M.: The Challenge of Implementing OASIS. Home Healthcare Nurse, 1998; 16(12):806–812.

Sitzman, K.: Tips for using OASIS. Home Healthcare Nurse, 1998; 16(8):561.

Sperling, R.: How OASIS relates to the Medicare 485. Home Healthcare Nurse, 1999; 17(2):82–85.

Sperling, R.: What's this OASIS, Anyway? Home Healthcare Nurse, 1998; 16(6):373–374.

Wellmark Fiscal Intermediary: Medicare Guide to Billing for HHAs. pp. 1–2. Des Moines, IA, Wellmark, Inc, 1997.

Wellmark Fiscal Intermediary: Medicare Guide to Billing for HHAs. pp. 13–20. Des Moines, IA, Wellmark, Inc, 1996.

Wilkinson, J. M.: Nursing Diagnosis and Intervention Pocket Guide, 6th edition. Menlo Park, Addison–Wesley Co, 1995.

Yuan, J. R.: Using Standards and Guidelines in Your Daily Practice. Home Healthcare Nurse, 1998; 16(11):753–759.

The Visit

7

This chapter discusses visit preparation, the visit, and postvisit activities. Each visit must be goal oriented and planned. The previsit activities include a review of the client's plan of care, a visit agenda, a check of necessary supplies and a verification of the appointment and directions to the home with the client.

Review the plans of care for all of your clients. Organize your schedule for the week based on the prioritization of the clients and their needs. Keep your clinical supervisor informed about your schedule.

PREVISIT ACTIVITIES

Plan your visits so they do not conflict with the other staff members' visits to the same client. That is one of the advantages of verifying your visits with the client beforehand. Frequently, clients will forget that they have another appointment scheduled at the same time you are coming. If you are seeing a client on Monday, Wednesday, and Friday, you can verify the Wednesday appointment when you see the client on Monday. It is wise to verify the Monday visit by phoning the client on Sunday evening or Monday morning. You would be surprised how many changes occur over the weekend. For example, the client may be admitted to the hospital or may forget about your visit and make another appointment. You may save yourself a wasted trip with a simple phone call.

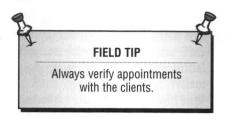

FIELD TIP

Always verify appointments
with the clients.

Supplies. Make sure that you have all of the supplies that you may need to use during the visit. Take extra supplies such as extra intravenous (IV) needles or vacutainer tubes in case you need more than one. When carrying extra supplies in your car, keep them in a clean, safe area, ensure that they are not outdated, and protect them from excess heat or cold. Many agencies will supply the field staff with styrofoam containers to protect the supplies. Take care that you do not carry excess supplies that become outdated and wasted. Everyone needs to help the agency remain financially solvent.

Since Medicare reimburses for supplies only as they are used, a balance needs to maintained between having sufficient supplies available in the home and not wasting them. Other payors may prefer to purchase the supplies and deliver them to the client's home. Those third-party payors may not be willing to reimburse the agency if you use its supplies.

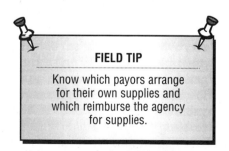

FIELD TIP

Know which payors arrange
for their own supplies and
which reimburse the agency
for supplies.

Any needed supplies must be included on the 485 form as the doctor's order or you will need to obtain an order from the doctor. It saves time if the initial plan of care (POC) includes any anticipated supplies, i.e., catheter supplies for the client with a Foley catheter. Listing a supply on the POC does not mean that it needs to be used, it just means that there is a potential need for the item.

When ordering supplies, specify the number and type of the supply. Use the generic name for the item. Medicare is more likely to reimburse for a generic item than for its more expensive counterpart. Sometimes the more expensive item may be needed to treat the client effectively. There must be documentation to justify the need for the more expensive supplies. The companies that supply those items employ representatives that can advise you on appropriate documentation that will help justify reimbursement. The company will usually list their toll-free phone number in the literature enclosed with the item or on the container.

If the doctor orders wound care for a specific number of days, you can take supplies just for those days. Most times, wound healing takes more than a few days, except in the case of an uncomplicated surgical wound. A good rule of thumb is to take a week's supply of dressings at a time. You will also want to make sure that there are sufficient supplies in the home in case a PRN (as needed) visit is necessary. Not only do you want to have supplies on hand for wound care or IV therapy in case of a PRN visit, but do not forget about extra catheter supplies for the client with a Foley catheter or tube feeding supplies for the client who is receiving tube feedings.

Be sure to charge for the supplies as you use them so they can be billed. You may think that it doesn't hurt to miss a 4 × 4 gauze pad once in awhile, but the cost of those few supplies can add up. At the first visit at which a roll of tape or bottle of saline is used, the item should be charged to the payor rather than charging a small amount with each visit. Medicare will reimburse for supplies used by the client while she/he is learning the procedure as long as it is justified in the documentation. Once the teaching is completed, the reimbursement is discontinued.

When blood is drawn for laboratory testing, the lab usually furnishes the needed supplies. Refer to the laboratory form for the appropriate vacutainer tube to be used. The initial of the tube stopper color will be found to the right of the desired procedure. It is wise to take a backup supply of needles and vacutainer tubes in case of an unsuccessful venipuncture. Additionally, make sure you have a biohazard container for the specimen.

Whether you have your own glucometer or use the agency's, keep it calibrated. Calibration should be done if:

>It has not been in use for a week or more
>After each battery change
>With each new bottle of reagent strips
>When the control test is out of range
>When the testing is done by a different operator.

A control test verifies that the test results are correct and the entire system is working properly. A control test should be run after calibration or any other time to check the accuracy of the system.

Teaching Preparation

Plan for client teaching before the visit. The teaching/learning process should be initiated at the time of the initial visit. The assessment phase should begin at this time. Assess the client's and caregiver's age, educational level, cognitive level, type of learner, level of motivation, level of understanding of condition, and emotional status. Also consider what the client needs to know and what she/he already knows.

Since most of the individuals that you will be teaching are adults, a review of characteristics of adult learners is in order. Adult learners tend to be self-directed, relate desired competencies to current competencies, value and expect meaningful learning experiences, and prefer interactive educational approaches. Because they are self-directed, you can provide adult learners with resources to obtain information and they will tend to pursue the learning experience. Motivation for learning is enhanced when the learners help to define their own learning objectives. Since they relate the desired competencies with competencies that they already possess, it helps if you have assessed their current competencies and can relate the learning to the clients' past experiences.

Because they value and expect meaningful learning experiences, learners should be provided with information about how the content will help them with their illness. This information will motivate them to learn the new content. Adapt instructional approaches to address the client's concerns and goals. Adults learn best through demonstrations, case situations, or actual experiences. Since they prefer interactive educational approaches, getting them actively involved in the learning experience improves their retention of the information. Provide a supportive learning environment that will foster active participation. Provide the client with encouragement and authentic feedback. In other words, let the client know what is learned correctly and what needs improvement.

All of us have varying styles of learning. The basic styles are auditory, visual, and kinetic. Most of us learn best through a combination of these three styles with one being more dominant than the others. If you combine these styles when teaching clients, their retention will be greater.

Studies demonstrate that learner recall more than doubles if the learning content is seen and heard. It more than triples if the content is seen and heard and the learner puts the information into action. Using this information should tell you that if you provide written handouts, learning will be more effective than if you just tell clients the information. If you review the information with the client and family along with providing written information and then have them put the learning into practice by having them repeat the information or practice the procedure, the retention is even greater.

When assessing the client for learning keep in mind that your teaching needs to be adapted to any physical problems, such as poor eyesight or hearing or impaired physical mobility. The client's culture, primary language, and level of anxiety are also factors that need to be considered when teaching.

Non-compliance is a favorite term used in health care when the client is perceived as not being interested in cooperating in his/her treatment. Non-compliance implies that the client is hopeless. Before labeling the client, look at what might be preventing the client from cooperating.

What is the client's motivation?
Is the client physically and mentally able to follow the instructions?

What are the external constraints to instructions such as lack of money?

What is the client's previous experience with health care?

Is the client experiencing anxiety or family problems that interfere with compliance?

It may be that you will have to assist the client with some of these issues before she/he will be ready to deal with his/her own health issues.

Once client and family learning needs have been assessed, the learning goals can be identified and the plan formulated. Begin by listing the client's learning needs. Then prioritize the needs. Involve the client and family in the planning phase. This is an effective way of motivating the client to participate in the learning process. Write out the learning goals for the client in clear terms, including the expected outcome date. These goals provide a basis for evaluating the client's progress. They also help others who are sharing in the teaching responsibilities to promote continuity.

Once you have determined what needs to be taught, you can prepare your teaching plans for the upcoming visit, including preparation of the teaching tools. There are brochures that can be purchased in bulk to be used to reinforce your teaching. There are some publications developed to assist the home health professional teach. They contain handouts that can be copied to give to the client. These publications will indicate if you have their permission to copy and use them as handouts. You can also make your own handouts. When the client is learning a skill such as checking his or her blood sugar, it helps to have the steps listed to cue the client while performing the procedure. This also reassures him/her that a step will not be forgotten.

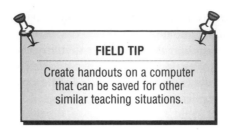

FIELD TIP

Create handouts on a computer that can be saved for other similar teaching situations.

THE VISIT

Upon arrival, introduce yourself if this is your first visit. Greet the client and family members by their formal names unless otherwise requested. Many people feel more comfortable being addressed by their first name but that is their option to choose. It is probably not necessary to remind you not to use names such as "grandpa," "dear," or "sweety."

Begin by assessing the client's status in all areas with a focus on his/her identified needs and goals. The assessment needs to include not only client needs and abilities but safety issues and any new problems. It is expected that the visit will take between 30 and 60 minutes. A visit less than 30 minutes is of questionable effectiveness.

Time Management

Time management skills will help you organize your overall schedule and visits. The key to managing your schedule is planning. Start by making a list of everything that needs to be done for the week. Include lunch breaks, meetings, and other appointments. Estimate the amount of time needed to perform each task.

Prioritize each item. If time is really tight, examine activities that can be combined. For example, can you make phone calls or document while eating lunch? Do not be a martyr by skipping lunch. You need that time to refresh yourself. You will think and function more effectively if you take the time to eat.

Delegate appropriate functions to others. The LPNs may be looking for visits to fill out their schedules. Allow reasonable time frames for completing each activity and some extra time to provide for unforeseen delays. Crossing off each completed function helps you see where you are in the schedule and gives you a sense of accomplishment. After planning your overall schedule for the week, plan for each individual visit. Block out time in your schedule for planning for each visit. Planning will help ensure that you do not forget an activity.

Identify and minimize or eliminate time wasters. No matter how well organized the agency office, it is easy to become involved in unnecessary conversations. Make a list of items that need to be done in the office so they can be completed quickly. This will help you make your office time more efficient. If you find that you are not able to control the interruptions at the office, consider completing your chart entries somewhere else. Some other quiet areas for charting are your home, a restaurant, public library, or a park. Keep in mind to maintain confidentiality of the client records.

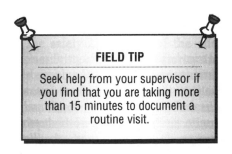

FIELD TIP

Seek help from your supervisor if you find that you are taking more than 15 minutes to document a routine visit.

Observations

Appendix A reviews observations that should be included when assessing and documenting conditions related to the various body systems. Your assessments must be consistent during each visit so you are able to observe early changes in the client's condition. You are more likely to detect changes because you are seeing the client on a more regular basis than even the doctor. The doctor and the payor expect that one of the major benefits of home health visits is to help prevent complications or detect early signs of complications so they can be treated early and prevent hospitalization.

To continue your ability to perform skilled observations, you need to remain up to date on information about the disease process and its complications. Keeping up to date requires constant pursuit of the latest information through journals, seminars, in-service sessions, and workshops. Medical information is considered to be out of date when it is over 5 years old. This implies that you need to constantly keep yourself up to date. You cannot completely depend on the information that you acquired in your basic program. That information is a valuable foundation, but you need to keep building on that foundation. Each agency should maintain a current library of resource materials for the field staff, but the staff professionals need to also subscribe to journals in their specialty areas.

If a client is admitted for services with a more uncommon condition, the tendency is for everyone to seek out information about that condition. The danger is when the client has a common condition such as diabetes mellitus, we feel that we already have all of the up-to-date information and do not seek further resources. The agency can help by providing in-service sessions, but do not be satisfied by depending totally upon the agency to keep you current. Additionally, keep your agency management informed about in-service presentations that would be helpful in your practice.

One complication that most, if not all, of your clients are prone to develop is infection. Protection against infection is more effective at home than in a structured facility but that doesn't mean that we can relax our infection control practices.

The most likely types of infection experienced by the home care client are of the urinary, respiratory, and integumentary systems. Clients who are prone to develop urinary tract infections are those with Foley catheters, fecal incontinence, dehydration, diabetes mellitus, cerebrovascular accident (CVA), multiple sclerosis, or a spinal cord injury. Clients prone to develop respiratory tract infections are those with prolonged immobility, obesity, dehydration, malnutrition, chronic respiratory or cardiovascular disease, or immunosuppression. Clients prone to develop skin infections are those who are immobile, obese, dehydrated, malnourished, those who have poor hygiene, diabetes mellitus, poor circulation, anemia, or those who use corticosteroids.

When assessing the client, you need to consider not only the client's diagnoses but also all potential complications. For example, the client with cardiovascular disease can develop congestive heart failure. Therefore in addition to assessing vital signs, heart sounds, and circulation, you need to be assessing for edema and auscultating the lung fields.

If your client has diabetes mellitus, you need to be assessing just about all of the body systems. You may be providing therapy services for a client who had a CVA. In addition to observing the client's progress in mobility or managing activities of daily living, you need to be assessing the client's vital signs and their orientation, especially if you are the only skilled service providing care.

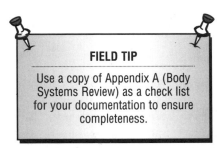

FIELD TIP

Use a copy of Appendix A (Body Systems Review) as a check list for your documentation to ensure completeness.

Skilled Interventions

Like skilled observations, you need to remain current with your psychomotor skills. The more you use each skill the more proficient you become. Becoming involved with the professional organizations that represent your specialty can help you keep up with the latest standards.

Provide skilled interventions appropriate for the client's problems. Do not forget that observation and teaching are skilled interventions, in addition to procedures. Frequently, we describe our role more by the procedures we perform than by the skills that require critical thinking.

Chapter 5, Infection Control discusses how equipment used for procedures is handled. Some of this equipment is kept in the client's home during the course of treatment. Other equipment, such as a stethoscope, is carried by the nurse or therapist to be used from client to client. Infection control practices need to be used on a regular basis.

CLINICAL PATHWAYS

Clinical pathways are gaining popularity in home health care. These programs are developed to lay out a standard program for clients with similar conditions. A clinical pathway is a sequence of processes and events that is designed to move the client toward expected outcomes. The pathways contain standards for care and disease- or discipline-specific outcome measurements. They also contain a documentation system for each discipline involved in the care.

The program is designed to save time for each discipline involved and avoid duplication of services. It is organized so that it can be individualized to meet the needs of each client. The educational plans are in manageable segments, specific to each visit. The program allows for consistency in care, teaching, and documentation among all of the skilled staff. Some client conditions that lend themselves to clinical pathways are diabetes mellitus, arthritis, total hip replacements, asthma, and chronic obstructive lung disease.

Complementary Therapy

When providing skilled care, keep in mind that the client may be using some complementary therapy too. Complementary therapy, also known as alternative therapy includes prayer, massage, herbal therapy, acupressure, relaxation, imagery, distraction techniques, aromatherapy, and therapeutic touch.

Some of these therapies may enhance the medical treatment, others may not help but are harmless, and others may be harmful. You need to be familiar with these therapies or at least be familiar with resources for information to be used when you have a client using them. Some of these therapies may be culturally based.

If it is not interfering with the medical treatment, you can help the client combine the complementary therapy with the medical treatment. Even if there are no physical benefits, frequently clients receive an emotional benefit from these therapies. If the client is using herbs, make sure that they are compatible with the client's medications. The client needs to be alerted if there is a harmful drug interaction. If the therapy can cause harm, the client also needs that information. The doctor also needs to be informed that a form of complementary therapy is being used.

Pain Management

Pain management is an important skill used by nurses and therapists. Clients with chronic pain, such as back pain and cancer pain, especially need this assistance. For chronic pain, the pain assessment should include its location, intensity, quality, and frequency and how it is relieved. The success of the pain management regimen can be tracked if all of these elements are addressed in the documentation on a weekly basis. Much success has been achieved with pain control when the client has been taught to manage his/her own pain program.

Functional Limitation Management

All home health professionals play a part in managing functional limitations. The disciplines involved in the care are going to depend on the cause of the limitations. Some clients require the care of more than one or all of the disciplines. The CVA client provides a good example. All of the disciplines need to work together and maintain frequent communication so there is not a duplication of services. All of the skilled staff members need to evaluate the client for functional limitations and to determine the appropriate therapy.

The occupational therapist (OT) will assess the client in his/her home to determine the extent of the environmental barriers and functional limitations. The OT will plan therapeutic exercises and adaptive equipment to help the client achieve optimal independence in activities of daily living (ADL) and home management.

The physical therapist (PT) will evaluate the client's mobility in the home environment. The PT assesses for barriers such as doorways and stairs and then plans an exercise program to increase mobility and overcome the barriers. The exercise program is also designed to help the client to eventually leave home.

The nurse will supervise the nursing assistant to ensure safe transfers and mobility of the client. If a therapist is not involved in the care, the nurse is responsible to supervise and teach the family caregiver how to safely assist the client with mobility and transfers.

The speech-language pathologist (SLP) will assess for the client's ability to swallow and communicate. The SLP will design a program of exercises to assist the client with these activities.

Maintenance therapy, which may be required to maintain function and prevent regression, does not always qualify for reimbursement. But there are situations in which the skills and judgment of a physical or occupational therapist are required to provide the services. A maintenance program may be instituted if, after evaluation, attempted therapy, and teaching, it is found that it is unlikely that the client's level of function can be restored to the same level as before services were required, but that it is likely that the client's level of functioning will regress without services. The potential danger to the client and the need for the skills of a therapist must be clearly documented.

Other Interventions

Venipunctures used to be considered a skilled service for reimbursement but that is no longer true. The client's care still could involve a venipuncture, and the visit will be reimbursed if an approved skilled intervention is provided at the same time. Some laboratories will provide technicians to draw blood for homebound clients for a nominal fee, if skilled visits are not justified.

When drawing blood for laboratory analysis, make sure you know how the sample needs to be handled. First, use the appropriate universal precautions for handling blood samples. All specimens must be labeled with the client's name, number, date, time drawn, and the initials of the person who drew the sample. Some samples need to be delivered within a particular period of time from when it is drawn, so you need to plan your visit accordingly. Find out if the specimen requires icing so you will have the proper supplies.

Intramuscular and subcutaneous injections can be reimbursed as a skilled intervention, at least for a limited period of time. The documentation needs to indicate that the injection is reasonable and necessary. If injections are required for an extended period of time, it is expected that the client or family caregiver will be taught how to handle the procedure. The injection will continue to be considered reimbursable only if the client or caregiver is not able to handle the injection, e.g., the client is blind, the family member has Alzheimer's disease.

Sometimes the client is able to administer his/her own injection as long as the syringes are prefilled. Prefilling syringes is not normally considered a reimbursable skill, but can be billed as a home health aide service if the client requires at least one skilled visit every 60 days, visits for prefilling syringes do not exceed every one to two weeks, and the client is not capable of filling the syringes. Some pharmacies provide the service of prefilling syringes so skilled visits would not be necessary.

Tube feedings and maintenance of the tube are reimbursable as a skilled service. Nasopharyngeal and tracheal suctioning and care are also reimbursable. Again, the intent is that these skills will eventually be taught to the client or family caregiver.

Wound care and IV therapy are two of the major nursing skills provided in home care. There is probably more wound care provided in the home now than in the hospital, considering the rapidity of hospital discharges. Intravenous antibiotic therapy at home is continually increasing in its popularity; IV therapy is reimbursable, but the antibiotic usually must be paid for by another payor. Catheter care for client's with a Foley catheter is also a reimbursable skilled service.

Dialysis treatments, especially the peritoneal type, could be covered in the home situation, however, if the client is receiving hemodialysis at a dialysis center, Medicare will not pay both the center and the home care agency. There are occasions when the dialysis client is receiving home health services for another diagnosis such as for an open wound, and these services would be reimbursed.

Chemotherapy may be a needed skilled home health service. The nurses providing the chemotherapy must be certified to provide the therapy safely.

Some psychiatric nursing services provided in the home care setting can be reimbursed by Medicare. The nurse providing those services must have special psychiatric training and/or experience beyond the basic registered nurse's education.

Management and evaluation of the plan of care was discussed earlier as a skilled service. The nurse or therapist is responsible for observation of the client's condition for possible modification of treatment or initiation of additional medical procedures until the client's treatment regimen is essentially stabilized. The nurse or therapist will also supervise the unskilled care being rendered to ensure that the care is achieving its purpose.

Teaching

The most important service that you can offer the client is your teaching skills. The main objective of teaching is to help the client and family become as independent as possible, as soon as possible. It is remarkable how well most clients and their family members can master the information and skills needed for them to become independent. There is some content that is taught in the hospital before the client is discharged that may need reinforcement. At least the amount of retention of the content needs to be assessed.

Consider physiologic and psychologic deficits in the client when teaching. If the client has problems with sight, provide printed materials in large (1-inch) black print. If the client has trouble concentrating, plan lessons that are no longer than 15 to 20 minutes. The teaching content should be taught at least two grade levels below the client's formal educational level. If the client or caregiver can comprehend the lesson and has the ability to recall the content, she/he will be motivated to learn more.

The more that you involve the client and family in the planning process, the more motivated she/he will be to learn. Begin the teaching with what the client already knows about the subject. Break the content down into manageable segments. This helps the learner find his/her bearings.

Take advantage of "learning moments." When the client or family member recognizes that she/he has a learning need and asks a question, take the time to teach rather than putting it off for another time. You can always reinforce that teaching at a later time. Relate the teaching material to the client's prior experience. Move from simple concepts to the more complex material.

Avoid deficiencies that interfere with learning. It is confusing if essential information is meshed with trivial facts or if too much information is given. Insufficient repetition of the material and use of terms that are too medically oriented will inhibit learning. The client's learning should be evaluated throughout the process to be sure the client is actually keeping up. Make sure that the client's illness is not interfering with learning. If the client is experiencing pain or nausea when you are trying to teach, chances are she/he will be focusing on the discomfort rather than what is being taught.

The sooner the client can apply the information the better. If the content is a cognitive type of information, have the client or caregiver repeat the information or explain it in his/her own words. If the content is psychomotor, have him/her give a return demonstration. Break the content down into segments. Do not try to teach too much at one time. Try to remember back to when you first learned some of these skills. It took a lot of practice to master the skill. The same will be true for the client.

At the next visit, have the client review the information from the prior visit before moving on to new content. Give him/her positive feedback to provide motivation. The client and caregiver need to know what should be corrected as well as what is being done correctly.

Take care about the terms that you use while teaching. When using medical terms, make sure the client understands their meaning. Providing a handout with a word list is very helpful. Avoid using acronyms. We get so used to using medical jargon that we forget that other people do not know the meaning of these terms. Use common terms as much as possible. Keep in mind that frequently clients will not ask you to clarify the meaning of the word because they do not want to appear dumb.

Observe the client's nonverbal behavior. It will help you pick up on indications of confusion. Ask the client open-ended questions to assess his/her understanding of the content. Rather than asking if the client understands the statement, ask him/her to explain the content. Propose a simulated situation, then ask the client to describe how she/he would respond.

Obtain feedback on how the client feels she/he is doing. You may have to adapt your teaching methods to make the teaching more effective. End the session by reviewing the content. Instruct the client about what can be practiced or reviewed before the next visit. Finish the session by documenting clearly. Be specific about what was taught and the client's response to the teaching session.

Subjects that need to be included in the teaching plan are new and changed medications, safety precautions, any new or changed diagnoses, and any exercises or procedures related to the client's therapy. The medication instructions need to include the medication's action, side-effects, drug interactions with other drugs and food, and precautions. When considering drug interactions, be sure to include over-the-counter drugs. You want to include content that will help the client learn to perform self-assessments and to know when it is appropriate to seek medical attention.

At the close of the visit review the client's progress with the client and family caregiver. It is wise to complete the visit documentation in the home as you can recall the details. As you document, you may think of other questions that need to be asked or information that needs to be shared with the client. If you document later, you may lose an opportune moment to help the client. Documentation is discussed in depth in Chapter 4. Be sure to include the client's response to services, progress toward goals, and the homebound status in your documentation. Confirm the next scheduled visit with the client and family before leaving.

POST VISIT ACTIVITIES

Take the time to evaluate the client's progress and any changes that should be made in the plan of care. During the postvisit time, communicate changes, make referrals, and replenish supplies. Communicate changes in the HHA care plan to the nursing assistant and the client. Any significant changes in the client's condition need to be communicated to the physician, the clinical supervisor, and the payor's case manager (if involved). Any other professionals involved in the client's care should be informed of any changes.

Investigate and contact any needed referral sources that you identified during the visit. Implementing referrals may have to include obtaining a physician's order or third-party payor approval. The goal of home care is to help the client and family become as independent as possible in managing the care. This management would include contacting referral sources. Therefore, the client will become independent sooner if you guide the client while she/he is obtaining the referral rather than making the referral yourself.

Begin your plan for the next visit. Arrange for any supplies that will be needed for the next visit. The supplies should include not only supplies for procedures, such as a dressing change, but also teaching supplies. Do not forget to charge for the supplies that were used during the visit.

References

Blanchard, L., Gill, G., and Williams, E.: Guidelines and Documentation Requirements for Social Workers in Home Health Care; Chapters 3 & 8. Silver Spring, MD: National Association of Social Workers, 1991.

Health Care Financing Administration: Home Health Agency Manual (HIM-11) Chapter II, Coverage of Services, Sec 200, pp. 11–24. Washington, D.C., Department of Health and Human Services. 1996.

Glasser, C. R.: Managing Functional Limitations. Home Health FOCUS, 1998; 4(12):89.

Knowles, M.: The Modern Practice of Adult Education. New York Association Press, 1970.

Long, C. O., Ismeurt, R. L., White, P. A.: Preventing Drug Interactions in the Home: A Five-Step Approach for Client Teaching. Home Healthcare Nurse, 1999; 17(2):106–112.

Management and Evaluation of a Care Plan. The Beacon Homecare FOCUS Series, pp. 1–16. Mequon, WI, Beacon Health, 1996.

Martin, J. P.: Home Care Orientation Manuel. CA Association for Health Services at Home. Sacramento, 1995.

Mason, J. E., and Hansen, J. F.: Teaching and Learning: An Overview, pp. 1–10. Patient Teaching Loose-leaf Library. Springhouse Corp., Springhouse, PA, 1991.

Olsten Health Services: Training and Development, OHM/Introduction to Medicare SSG, 1/97, pp 4-3 to 4-6. Melville, NY, Olsten Health Services, 1997.

Olsten Health Services: Transitional Nurses Orientation Learner Guide, Chapter 2, 4–2 to 4–4. Melville, NY, Olsten Health Services, 1997.

Pearson, M., and Wessman, J.: Gerogogy in Patient Education. Home Healthcare Nurse, 1996; 14(8):631–636.

Perry, S., and Shipes, E.: Collecting Assessment Data, pp. 11–30. Patient Teaching Loose-leaf Library. Springhouse Corp., Springhouse, PA, 1991.

Rimmer, L. M.: What Every Home Healthcare Nurse Should Know About Complementary Therapy. Home Healthcare Nurse, 1998; 16(11):760–764.

Rowe, P., and Wells, E. A.: Planning for Teaching, pp. 31–42. Patient Teaching Loose-leaf Library. Springhouse Corp., Springhouse, PA, 1991.

Rowe, P., and Tackenberg, J. N.: Implementing the teaching plan, pp. 43–48. Patient Teaching Loose-leaf Library. Springhouse Corp., Springhouse, PA, 1991.

Sherry, D.: Time Management Strategies of the New Home Care Nurse. Home Healthcare Nurse, 1996; 14(9):718–720.

Sitzman, K.: Tips for Using OASIS. Home Healthcare Nurse, 1998; 16(8):561.

Sperling, R.: How OASIS relates to the Medicare 485. Home Healthcare Nurse, 1999; 17(2):82–85.

Stempel, J.: Pain Management in Terminal Illness. Home Health FOCUS, 1997; 4(3):17–19.

Case Manager Responsibilities

8

This chapter discusses the various case management responsibilities of the home health nurse or therapist. The discussion focuses on how these responsibilities vary in home health from those in acute and long-term nursing and therapy. See Table 8–1 for an overview of the case management responsibilities.

Some home health agencies use all of their nurses and therapists as case managers, whereas others may use only select professionals as case managers. No matter the type of system at your agency, all of the professionals will be expected to share some of these responsibilities.

The case manager is responsible for the overall coordination of services for the client, maintenance of an up-to-date client chart, supervision of home health aides (HHAs) and licensed vocational/practical nurses (LVNs, LPNs), discharge planning, and recertification of the case when appropriate. Usually, the individual who admits the client to the agency services is the one who manages the care. That professional will have a more thorough understanding of the client and the client's environment, and therefore, will have a better understanding of the individual's strengths and weakness.

The responsibilities involved with the management of the client's care include the conduct of comprehensive assessments and the setting of client goals. Additionally, the case manager designs the teaching plans and interventions and plans the visits.

Table 8–1	RESPONSIBILITIES OF THE CASE MANAGER

Development of the plan of care
Coordination of client services
Maintenance of the client's chart
Supervision of HHAs and LPN/LVNs
Discharge planning
Case recertification

PHYSICIAN COMMUNICATION

To provide coordination of the client's care, effective communication and collaboration are required. First and foremost, the case manager needs to keep the physician informed about the client's progress toward his/her goals. Doctor's orders are needed to cover the plan of care (POC) for the client and any changes in the POC before they are implemented. Each order must specify the modality or treatment, the discipline involved, and the frequency and duration of visits. Changes that require a doctor's order include either an increase or a decrease in services. In other words, before increasing or decreasing the frequency of visits, doctor's orders must be obtained. The agency must have signed orders on file prior to billing for those services. Fiscal intermediaries (FI) report that the main reasons for denial of home health claims are no doctor's orders and missing documentation.

In structured facilities, the nurse does not need a doctor's order to assign an aide to care for a client, but this order is required in home health. The case manager can obtain these change orders by telephone or fax, depending on the doctor's preference. The more skilled you become in determining frequencies and durations, the fewer change orders you will have to obtain.

Each professional discipline is responsible to obtain it's own change orders. Even when there is no need for updated orders, the physician needs to be informed about the client's progress. This can be done with a brief call to the physician's office nurse. When you are expecting a return call from the doctor or from one of the physician's office staff, be sure that you keep the clinical supervisor informed in case the call comes in when you are out of the office. There is nothing more frustrating to a doctor than to return a phone call and find no one in the office who seems to know why she/he was contacted. That situation is not an effective way of maintaining a positive image for the agency.

It is helpful to improve communications with the physician by making occasional visits to his/her office when the client has an appointment. This is especially beneficial when the client requires long-term care or when a client has an extensive or complicated wound.

All communications with the physician or the office should be documented even when the outcome is unsuccessful. If the communication occurs through one of the doctor's staff members, record the name of that person.

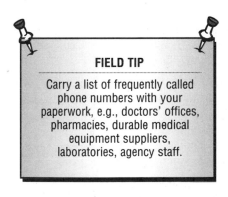

FIELD TIP

Carry a list of frequently called phone numbers with your paperwork, e.g., doctors' offices, pharmacies, durable medical equipment suppliers, laboratories, agency staff.

PAYOR REPRESENTATIVES

The case manager also needs to maintain contact with the representative (case manager) of the payor agency that is involved in the client's care. If the client's care is totally reimbursed by Medicare, there would not be another case manager involved; however, if all or part of the care is reimbursed by insurance, a health maintenance organization (HMO), or another payor, each service covered by that payor must be approved before the visits are made.

It is wise to obtain those approvals in writing via fax before implementing the visits. Some payors have been known to deny payment if the approvals are not in writing. Sometimes, the nurse or therapist may have some difficulty convincing the payor representative that particular visits are needed. If you feel that you have not obtained appropriate approval for the client, consult with your supervisor. Frequently, you or your supervisor can request to speak to the payor's manager, who will most likely be a nurse or physician. It always helps to know the credentials of the individual with whom you are speaking. That information will help you know how much explanation about the client's condition is needed for the payor's case manager to understand your request. Even if the payor representative is a registered nurse (RN) or another professional, she/he may not be familiar with home health and may require education about some issues peculiar to home care.

Keep in mind that you are the client's advocate. You want to be reasonable in your requests for service approvals but you want to make sure that the client receives safe care by clearly communicating his/her needs. Provide a clear picture of the client's medical and home situation. Do not hesitate to make suggestions about services that can improve the client's outcome. Sometimes it helps to proceed with the approval that you are able to obtain even if you feel it will be inadequate. You can always call back later when you have more data to support your position. There are other times that you find that the original approval was sufficient. If the payor will not approve visits that you know are needed, be sure to ask for that denial in writing and that you also document the denial. There are times when a payor who is requested to put a denial in writing decides that some more home visits might be appropriate. Make sure that any additional visits are covered by the doctor's orders.

It is helpful to provide consistent and concise reports that keep the payor's representative up-to-date regarding the client's progress. The payor expects that the client is provided services in a timely fashion and to be kept informed about the client's care. Building a working relationship with the payor source will facilitate the client's progress toward his/her goals. Keep in mind that the case manager for the payor is under pressure to maintain a balance between meeting the client's needs for quality care and keeping the costs of the care as low as possible. She/he will appreciate your cooperation in this endeavor.

HOME HEALTH TEAM

The home health case manager needs to maintain knowledge of the client's progress toward all goals. This involves contact with all disciplines providing nursing and therapy services.

Are the appropriate disciplines involved in the client's care? The case manager needs to be familiar with the scope of practice for each discipline so appropriate referrals can be made. The clinical supervisor can help determine if the referral should be made.

A social work referral may be in order if social or emotional problems are interfering with the effective treatment of the client's medical condition or rate of recovery. Treatment of the client's family would not be considered reimbursable except if that treatment is reasonable and necessary in order to treat the client's condition. Social work services can make the difference between a successful course of treatment for the client and the need for rehospitalization or reinstitutionalization. The goal of home health social work services is to improve or maintain the social, emotional, functional, and physical health status of the client and to enhance the coping skills of the family or significant others.

Occupational therapy is an appropriate referral if the client has lost the ability to perform activities of daily living (ADL), home management activities, or play and leisure activities. The occupational therapist (OT) works with clients who have upper extremity or hand problems.

Physical therapy is appropriate when the client is in need of rehabilitation because of an inability to ambulate or transfer safely. This includes the need for improvement of balance, gait, or range of motion. The physical therapist (PT) will help family members learn to assist the client in mobilization and also help the client deal with musculoskeletal pain.

The role of speech language pathology services has not been appreciated until recently. Those services are appropriate if the client is experiencing difficulties swallowing or has difficulty communicating, either verbally, or with reading or writing.

Skilled nursing is appropriate when the client is in need of skilled observation, teaching, or intervention for a medical or surgical condition or injury. Some appropriate nursing interventions include wound care, intravenous therapy, medication administration, and urinary catheter care.

The case manager must consider several factors when coordinating the client's care, such as the need to continue the services of any disciplines into the next certification period, and the progress of the client and family caregiver in assuming more responsibility for the ADLs so that the nursing assistant services can be reduced or discontinued.

The client and family should be informed about the status of the services and anticipated discharge plans for each discipline. Clients need to be informed about discharge plans at least one visit prior to the discharge day. They must understand that the services of the certified nursing assistant (CNA) will be discontinued along with the discharge of the last professional discipline.

Maintaining communication between the field staff can be accomplished via phone, case communication notes, and weekly case conferences meetings. The nurse or therapist can keep informed about client's progress with ADLs through regular supervisory visits. The communication among the disciplines needs to be a two-way process. In other words, the case manager needs to keep the others informed about the client's progress or lack of progress.

The case manager is responsible for maintaining the client's chart, keeping it updated at all times. She/he has the ultimate responsibility to ensure that the charting remains in compliance with company policies, payor requirements, and state and federal regulations including Medicare conditions of participation. This responsibility involves updating medication sheets, care plans, recertifications, and supervisory visits. In addition to assuring that accurate visit notes are maintained, documentation of management and coordination aspects of the care need to be included. One example is the coordination of services from other agencies such as Meals on Wheels or housekeeping.

Any time the client is transferred to a different facility such as the hospital, even for a short period of time, this transfer needs to be documented and all disciplines caring for the client must be notified. Most agencies have a particular form that can be used for this purpose. This form is usually designed with multiple copies that can be distributed to all agency personnel involved in the client's care; the original copy is placed in the client's chart. Another time the case communication form is used is when the client dies. It is important to inform the field staff as soon as possible about transfers and deaths to save them from unnecessary trips and even more important to save them and the family from embarrassing moments.

CASE CONFERENCES

Case conferences are one of the major means for the home health staff to coordinate the care of the agency clients. There are various formats that can be used to present case conferences. Factors that can affect how they are organized are the size of the agency and the type of clients served by that agency.

Many agencies use more than one type of format for case conferences. When the agency is caring for a client with a very complicated case that involves nursing, one or two different therapists, and an aide, a case conference involving all of the disciplines to focus on the one client can promote a uniform progression toward common client goals. Another common format frequently used is a weekly case conference attended by the field staff to review the progress of clients who are due for recertification, those receiving wound care, and those receiving intravenous (IV) therapy. Additionally, any clients with special problems are discussed. Any given client is discussed at least one time per certification period; however, most clients are discussed more frequently.

If the agency is small, all of the field staff could meet together in one weekly case conference. In larger agencies, it is more efficient for each individual clinical supervisor to meet with his/her team. Because of the nature of home health, communication does not come easy; therefore, it is essential that all staff members make sure that they are present for the weekly case conferences. You will find that weekly attendance not only promotes continuity of care for the clients but is an opportunity for the staff to receive help solving special client care problems.

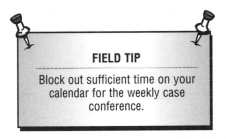

FIELD TIP

Block out sufficient time on your calendar for the weekly case conference.

SUPERVISION

Case managers who are RNs are expected to supervise the care rendered by LPNs and nursing assistants. Therapist case managers are expected to supervise therapy provided by aides and assistants. When an LPN is participating in the client's care, the RN is expected to provide a supervisory visit with the LPN present at least once a certification period. If the RN and LPN are sharing the visits and the RN sees the client on a regular basis, the supervisory visit can be made during one of the RN's visits without the LPN being present. The RN would obtain the client's and family's input about their satisfaction or lack of satisfaction with the services. Even if a visit with the LPN present is not required, an occasional visit to observe the LPN providing care is an opportunity to assess the nurse's skills and provide helpful feedback.

The Medicare Conditions of Participation (COP) require that supervisory visits for nursing assistant services occur at least every 14 days. Other payors have variations of this regulation. When case managing care paid for by different payors, you need to become familiar with their regulations.

The nursing assistant supervisory visits do not all have to be with the aide present, but at least one time during the certification period a supervisory visit must occur with the aide present. That does not mean that you do not have to maintain communication with the CNA(s) if you want to provide continuity of care for the client, especially if the aides are not included in the weekly case conferences. The aides need to know when changes have been made in the care plan and their input needs to be obtained about the client's progress. The case managers do not always appreciate the information that the CNAs can contribute about the client and family that could affect the client's progress. Keep in mind that the aide probably spends more time with the client and family than any of the other agency staff members. They are usually the first ones to recognize when the client is ready to progress from a sponge bath to a shower or when she/he is becoming too unstable to continue getting into a tub.

Frequently, the CNAs do not feel appreciated. The agency professionals can provide the support needed to encourage the nursing assistants and prevent high turnovers in the CNA positions. The support can be manifested by encouraging their feedback and providing them with information that will help them provide good care.

Communication can be fostered by arranging more frequent supervisory visits with the CNA present. Encourage the nursing assistant to contact you when they notice changes or have concerns. The case manager is responsible for auditing the CNA's visit notes at the time of the supervisory visit to make sure that the care plan is followed and no problems have arisen. CNAs are required to record on the client visit note and verbally report any changes that need immediate attention. However, if the change does not need to be addressed right away, they will usually document it and may or may not report it later. Sometimes nursing assistants assume that the RN or therapist is going to read their documentation immediately. Encourage them to keep you informed about important documentation, in case you do not have the opportunity to read the notes right away.

When supervising the employee observe him/her for skill performance. Is the employee reliable? Is the care plan followed? Are the principles of universal precautions and bag technique being followed? Most important, does the employee treat clients and family members and their property with respect? Can the aide deal with emergencies appropriately?

Make a point of providing feedback for the CNAs. Do not just focus on areas that need improvement. Always balance those areas with positive feedback. If you avoid giving corrective feedback, you can not expect the CNAs to make improvements. On the other hand, the nursing assistants also need the positive input to reinforce their positive behavior. Even if they know that they are doing well, positive feedback encourages them to continue doing a good job.

Are the client and family satisfied with the CNA services? The supervisory visit is an opportune time to involve the client and family in planning the care by obtaining their input about any needed changes.

One of the greater challenges regarding supervisory visits is to track them so they are performed on schedule. Some agencies track these visits on the computer, but you cannot always depend on the computer's accuracy. The data in the computer are only as good as the individual who inputs the data. Therefore, the case manager is the one who is ultimately responsible to track the visits.

It helps to initiate a calendar for each client when she/he is admitted to the agency's services. Plug in the anticipated supervisory visits for the certification period. Be sure to alter the visit dates on the calendar if you happen to make the visits ahead of the scheduled date. If you make the supervisory visit a couple of days early, it is acceptable but you then need to alter your calendar so the next visit takes place no later than within the required 14 days. Of course, the next challenge is to remember to check each client's calendar so you don't miss the visit. Keep in mind that supervisory visits alone are not reimbursible by Medicare except when combined with a skilled service. So if possible arrange the visits to combine both objectives.

Documentation of the supervisory visit should include the staff member who is being supervised, his/her title, and if that person was present. If the staff member was present, include what tasks were observed, the employee's competency in performance of the skills, and any training or instruction provided. You also want to include any changes in the care plan, if the client was notified about the changes, and if the client/family are satisfied with the care. Do not forget to include the client's continuing needs and progress toward the goals.

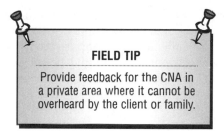

FIELD TIP

Provide feedback for the CNA in a private area where it cannot be overheard by the client or family.

CARE PLANS

The LPN follows the same plan of care that is followed by the RN. The case manager is responsible for delegating the LPN's assignments appropriately, based on the state's nurse practice act's definition of the LPN/LVN's scope of practice and the agency's job description. The directions for the LPN and any RN participating in the client care need to be complete, understandable, logical, and clear, and indicate their importance. It is helpful to obtain feedback from the nurses to be sure they did understand the directions. You need to follow up on these directions to be sure there was no misunderstanding and that they were carried out without any problems. You also need to keep informed about the client's response to the care rendered by the other nursing staff.

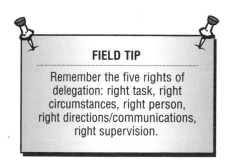

FIELD TIP

Remember the five rights of delegation: right task, right circumstances, right person, right directions/communications, right supervision.

The care plans that are required for the nursing assistants need to be written by the RN or therapist for the specific client with clear directions so the CNA does not have to guess about what should be included in the client care. The nursing assistants need to know exactly when each skill is to be performed. An as needed (PRN) order should never be used for the CNA care plan. If there is a skill, such as a shampoo, that the client would not want with each visit, the directions can specify that it would be done according to the client's preference.

The care plan needs to include only the skills permitted under state law and according to the agency's job description. When ordering any measurements of vital signs, the orders must include the expected parameters for those signs and the directions to notify the office if the client's vital signs fall outside the parameters.

The type of bath needs to be specified. If the client has a sponge bath ordered but progresses to a shower, the care plan must be changed accordingly. The Medicare COPs indicate that the CNA is there to provide personal care. There may be other activities performed by the nursing assistant during the visit, such as a meal preparation but this should not be the only reason the CNA is providing care. One Medicare intermediary may interpret this regulation differently from another. One may expect to see that the aide provides a bath or shower with each visit, while the other may consider that skin care, oral care, and dressing assistance would qualify for reimbursement. You need to keep informed how the intermediary in your agency's region interprets the regulations.

The care plan needs to specify the client's level of activity and any safety factors involved in the client's care. Additionally, any assistance for elimination or intake/output needs to be included.

If any meals need to be prepared and served to the client, the diet needs to be specified. Client allergies and if there is a DNR order are always recorded on the care plan. Any special precautions or instructions that must be reported should be included. Dates of updates and by whom they are made must be noted on the care plan. These updates need to be recorded on the original care plan in the client's chart and on the copy in the client's home folder.

RECERTIFICATION

The Medicare COPs require that the total plan of care is updated and reviewed by the physician and agency personnel as often as the severity of the client's condition requires but at least once every two months (57 to 62 days). The case manager is responsible for tracking the client's case so that the recertification process is instituted at the appropriate time. When the client is admitted to the agency services, record on the client's calendar the date that the process needs to begin in order to obtain a new signed plan of care before the beginning of the next certification period; usually that date is 45 days from the start of care.

Recently, the Health Care Financing Administration (HCFA) has indicated that the Outcome and Assessment Information Set (OASIS) assessment for recertification needs to be performed within the last 5 days (57 to 62 days) of the current certification period. This severely limits the recertification time frame but there are several issues that can be handled before that 5-day window. First, the client's case can be discussed at case conference to determine if it is appropriate to continue any skilled services. If not, then all of the skilled disciplines need to be discharged before the last day of the certification period. This includes the CNA services if any are being provided.

There may be one or two of the skilled services that are ready to discharge the client but one that needs to continue, which indicates that the case needs to be recertified. Depending on the agency's policies, the discipline for which continuing skilled services are required would usually be the one responsible for recertifying the case.

During the case conference, any changes in care and goals need to be determined. Once the need for recertification is identified, contact the physician to obtain the order to continue care. This order keeps the doctor informed about the client's status and provides orders to cover the time while you are waiting for the newly signed 485 form to return from the doctor's office. This is especially needed now that HCFA does not want the OASIS assessment completed until 5 days before the end of the certification period. The verbal order to continue care must be recorded in the client record and recorded on the 485 form for the physician's signature.

In addition to updating the client's problem list, goals, and orders to achieve the goals, all of the information on the 485 form needs to be updated. If you make a copy of the client's 485 form and update the information in red directly on the copy, the data entry clerk can accurately identify the needed changes. Consider the following questions:

1. Is the current attending physician recorded on the form?
2. Are the client's address and phone number current? (If the address has been changed, make sure that directions to the home are also current in the client record.)
3. Have the certification dates been changed? (The last day of the current period becomes the first day of the next certification period. The last day of the new period is two months from the first day.)

4. Has the client's payor been changed? (If so, insure that the proper verification and authorizations have been made. It is not unusual to discover that the client has changed their payor; for example, a client may move from Medicare to a HMO or vice versa in the middle of a certification period. If the appropriate authorizations from the current payor have not been obtained, the payor will not be responsible for the bills.)

5. Has the medication sheet been updated to reflect the client's current medications and dosages?

6. Are the dates of onset or exacerbation of the diagnoses current?

7. Has the CNA care plan been reviewed, updated, signed, and dated?

8. Have the nursing assistant notes been reviewed for compliance with the care plan?

9. Are all supervisory visits documented and in compliance?

10. Are all services covered by signed physician orders?

During the recertification visit, perform a complete assessment of the client, including the OASIS assessment items. On the basis of that assessment, you will need to update the client's problem list, interventions, and goals. During the visit, it is wise to review the Patient Bill of Rights with the client and family, especially the information regarding the proper individual to call to resolve complaints.

Most agencies will have a form that summarizes the client's progress to be filled out after the recertification assessment of the client. This summary report is placed in the client's record; a copy must also be sent to the physician. This document includes the client's current condition, limitations, skilled services being provided, and progress toward goals. Also included are any new problems and goals.

Lastly, a calendar for the next certification period should be generated; mark anticipated supervisory visit dates and the date to assess for the next recertification, including the 5-day recertification window. All of the recertification paperwork needs to be submitted in a timely fashion so the new 485 form can be prepared and sent to the physican for signature.

DISCHARGE PLANNING

Ideally, discharge planning begins at the start of care. It is expected that the discharge plan will be shared with the client and family prior to the last visit. If the client's care is not going to be recertified, the last visit must be on the day before the last date in the certification period to be covered by the orders of the current certification period. The "to" date of the certification period means up to but not including that date. If recertified, the "to" date becomes the first day of the next period.

Each professional discipline documents his/her own discharge summary. The physician should be notified by phone of the discharge for verification of the physician's agreement. The discharge summary(s) is then mailed to the doctor for his/her signature. Make sure that any involved payor is notified of the discharge. Make sure that the discharge date covers all of the disciplines in the home, including the home health aide. For example, if you make the discharge visit on Tuesday afternoon but the CNA is to make one more visit on Wednesday morning, make the discharge date to cover Wednesday. Otherwise, the last nursing assistant visit will not be reimbursed.

When making the last visit, assess the client to insure that she/he has reached the goals. The last assessment includes some more OASIS items that must be addressed. Review any instructions with the client and family to be sure there are no questions. Observe the client or caregiver perform any new skills. Review any remaining concerns or questions. Explore any needs for referrals and help the client make the referrals as appropriate. If a CNA was providing services and the client still needs personal care services, explore some other options, such as private duty services. If needed, leave written instructions.

The discharge summary includes skilled services provided, the client's continuing care needs, instructions given, and referrals made. Additionally, a summary of the client's condition and services provided during the client's care is documented. Include which goals were met and which ones were not met. If a goal was not met, include an explanation of why it was not met. Finally what is the client's physical, emotional, mental, and functional condition at the time of discharge.

Occasionally, the client is discharged without the last home health professional's visit. Some examples of those instances include:

When the client is admitted to a hospital or skilled nursing facility

When it becomes evident that the client no longer meets the basic requirements for home health services, e.g., no longer homebound

When the client decides that she/he does not need the home health services.

The discharge summary still needs to be recorded.

If the client is admitted to the hospital, it does not mean an automatic discharge. Each agency will have policies to provide guidelines in the case of a hospital admission. Some agencies will automatically discharge the client upon admission to the facility while others allow a 2-week period in the facility before discharging the client. If the client develops a condition while hospitalized that further complicates the care, it might be better to discharge the client and then evaluate for readmission once the client returns home. The client cannot be recertified while in the hospital. This is another factor to consider when making the decision to discharge. If it is close to the end of the certification period, it may be better to discharge the client. If the client is discharged and readmitted, the certification period dates are changed to coinside with the new start of care date.

When the client is transferred to a facility without being discharged from home health services, a short OASIS form is completed. You will want to keep track of the client. The client and family may appreciate a courtesy visit to the client in the hospital. Of course this would not be a billable visit. Some agencies may have a staff member visit all of the agency's clients who may be in the hospital. It also helps to maintain contact with the hospital's discharge planner to be sure she/he remembers that the individual is the agency's client. These contacts also help you keep up with the client's progress. When resuming care after discharge from the hospital, you should make a comprehensive assessment and update the plan of care.

CALL RESPONSIBILITIES

On-call systems vary from agency to agency. The determining factors are the size of the agency and the number of clients on service. Larger agencies have administrative RNs handle the calls when the office is closed and delegate the visits to the appropriate staff member. Smaller agencies may have the staff nurses handle the incoming calls and make the necessary visits.

Home health agencies would not be able to function without the on-call participation of all field staff, especially the nurses and CNAs. There are routinely scheduled visits that need to be made on weekends and in the evenings. Some nurses prefer to make the off-hour visits for their clients to provide better continuity of care. Others feel that they need the time off to refresh themselves. In addition to the routine visits, there are admissions that need to be initiated in the evenings or on the weekend and there are PRN calls that need attention.

If you are having someone else make your visit, write clear instructions and client information. Include the client's name, number, address, and phone number. Additionally, give the client's diagnosis and clear orders for the visit; indicate if supplies are in the home and if the client has a do not resuscitate order. Give detailed directions to the home and the time required to make the visit. It is helpful for the employee making the visit to have a copy of the notes from the prior visit. That gives the staff member an idea of the client's current condition.

If you are the staff member making the call, phone the client to verify the time of the visit. The client usually knows that the regular nurse or therapist will not be there but worries about who will be coming and if she/he will be coming at the usual time. If there is no verification call, the client can become so upset that the nurse or therapist will have to spend the first 10 minutes of the call helping the client calm down. A verification call is a courteous way to introduce yourself before the actual visit. It can also provide an opportunity to clarify the directions to the home. Remember to use extra safety precautions when making visits at night.

It is not always easy making PRN visits in the middle of the night, but the gratitude of the client and family makes up for the inconvenience. The administrative RN is responsible for screening the calls so unnecessary visits are kept to a minimum. If the family calls the agency in an emergency, such as a fall that caused a fractured hip, it is a waste of time to send out a nurse who would probably assess the client and call for an ambulance. The family needs to be instructed to call the ambulance themselves. Tell them that you will call back in a few minutes to make sure they were successful in contacting the paramedics.

There are other minor problems that can be dealt with on the phone with the client or family member. The individual who is screening the calls needs to make sure that the PRN visits are covered by doctor's orders. If there are no orders, the administrative RN needs to obtain them.

QUALITY ASSURANCE

At least quarterly, the agency professionals representing the scope of the services provided will review a sample of active and closed clinical records. The chart audits are done to determine if policies were followed while those services were provided. The home health professional staff are expected to participate in the agency's performance appraisal.

The agency will select particular identifiers to be examined that would indicate that the agency is in regulatory compliance. Client records are selected at random to be audited by the staff to verify the presence of each identifier. Some identifiers that could be included are:

Are the doctor's orders signed and dated?
Have supervisory visits been made every 14 days?

Is the client Bill of Rights signed?

Is the client's homebound status clearly documented?

Are the skilled services documented for each visit?

Is the client's progress toward goals recorded?

Has the client been informed about the discharge plan?

Have the client and family received instruction at each visit?

Is the HHA care plan being followed?

Professional staff members have found that auditing charts helps keep them up to date on home health regulations. Staff members who are new to home health especially benefit from this experience.

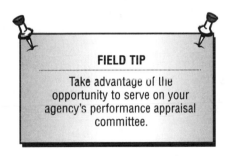

FIELD TIP

Take advantage of the opportunity to serve on your agency's performance appraisal committee.

References

A Homecare Therapist Guide to Medicare Service Delivery. The Beacon Homecare FOCUS Series, Medicare Reimbursement for Therapy Services, pp. 1–9. Mequon, WI, Beacon Health, 1996.

Czarnik, B.: Medicare Coverage Issues. Home Healthcare Nurse, 1997; 15(7):512–514.

Danks, S. A.: Building Relationships with Medicare Managed-Care Case Managers. Home Healthcare Nurse, 1999; 17(1):53–56.

Dreyer, C. J.: Home Health Aide Supervision: Care Plans and Supervisory Visits. Home Health FOCUS, 1998; 5(6):45.

Gorski, L. A.: Case Management: Collaboration is Essential. Home Health FOCUS, 1998; 5(5):38.

Harris, M. D.: Medicare and the Nurse. Home Healthcare Nurse, 1998; 16(11):732–736.

Harris, M.: The Physician as a Member of the Home Healthcare Team. Home Healthcare Nurse, 1998; 16(11):732–735.

Health Care Financing Administration: Home Health Agency Manual (HIM-11), Chapter II, Coverage of Services, Sec 200, pp. 11–24. Washington, D.C., Department of Health and Human Services, 1987.

Health Care Financing Administration: Home Health Agency Manual (HIM-11), Chapter II, Coverage of Services, Sec 200, pp. 11–24. Washington, D.C., Department of Health and Human Services, 1996.

Health Care Financing Administration: OASIS Implementation Manual, Attachment B. pp. 8.62–8.75. Washington D.C., Department of Health and Human Services, 1998.

Hilliard, L. S.: Manager's Corner: Innovative or Disintegrate. Home Care Nurse News, 1998; 5(6):1–2, 8.

Hogue, E. E.: Communications with Physicians (Handout). Burtonsville, MD, 1998.

Management and Evaluation of a Care Plan. The Beacon Homecare FOCUS Series, pp. 1–16. Mequon, WI, Beacon Health, 1996.

Martin, J. P.: Home Care Orientation Manual. California Association for Health Services at Home, Sacramento, 1995.

Medicare Bulletin #416, by bcc (Blue Cross Calif.) Fiscal Intermediary, Oxnard, CA, July 13, 1998, p. 13.

Medicare Reimbursement of Therapy Services. The Beacon Homecare FOCUS Series, pp. 1–9. Mequon, WI, Beacon Health, 1996.

Olsten Health Services: Training and Development, OHM/Introduction to Medicare SSG, 1/97, 3–3 to 3–10. Melville, NY, Olsten Health Services, 1997.

Olsten Health Services: Client Care Management for Hospital Alliance Home Health Agencies, Supervision, 10–6 to 10–8. Tampa, FL, Olsten Management Services, 1995.

Sperling, R.: How OASIS relates to the Medicare 485. Home Healthcare Nurse, 1999;17(2):82–85.

Stonerock, C.: Home Health Aides: Home Care's "Endangered Species." Home Care Provider, 1997; 2(1):15–17.

Touchard, B. M. and Berthelot, K.: Collaborative Home Practice: Nursing and Occupational Therapy Ensure Appropriate Medication Administration. Home Healthcare Nurse, 1999; 17(1):45–51.

Wellmark Fiscal Intermediary: Medicare Guide to Billing for HHAs, pp. 1–22. Des Moines, IA, Wellmark, Inc., 1997.

Ethical Issues 9

This chapter discusses ethical issues as they relate to home care. Issues such as confidentiality, conflicts of interest, client rights, and personal involvement will be examined. The basic ethical principles provide guidelines for home health professionals, just as they would for practitioners employed in structured facilities. However, the circumstances encountered in home care provide different challenges for maintaining ethical principles.

CONFIDENTIALITY

Confidentiality of Records

Confidentiality is one of those issues that poses special challenges to be considered in home health. The home care practitioner carries greater responsibility for maintaining confidentiality of client records than do professionals employed in structured facilities. In hospitals and skilled nursing facilities, client records remain in the facility. In home care, employees need to carry client information with them when providing services. Usually there is no need for home health personnel to carry a complete client record but some documents always need to be carried. There are some occasions when a practitioner will need to carry the complete chart, such as with a client admission. That record needs to be returned to the agency as soon as possible.

Home care employees are responsible for the security of any client documents in their possession. This responsibility needs to be kept in mind whether the documents are in the employee's car, home, or office or in the client's home. One basic principle that facilitates record security is to carry only the documents that are absolutely needed to provide client care. Documents containing detailed information about the client's condition should not be left in the home.

The employee's family needs to be instructed that any client records used at home are confidential and must be kept secure. Keep the records in a secure area and out of reach of children. When records are carried in the car, they must be locked up and out of sight. Preferably, they should be locked up in the trunk of the vehicle. If you do not have a trunk, they should be placed out of site, e.g., under the seat. Avoid leaving the records in the car when you are not making visits.

Never carry one client's documents into another client's home. You may think that no one else would look through your papers but you must be able to be assured that the records are secure. There are times during the visit when you might need to leave the records unattended, such as when changing the client's dressing. You could not testify that someone did not look at the documents when you were out of the room. Just carry in the record of the client you are visiting and leave the other clients' records locked in the vehicle.

Even in the agency office, security precautions must be used. When not in use, client documents should be locked in a desk or file. Over night, the most secure area for client records is locked up in the records room. Each agency needs to establish a system to keep track of client charts. You need to be familiar with and follow the agency policies regarding records.

As soon as you no longer are caring for a client, all documents that contain the client's information must be destroyed. The most secure procedure for that purpose is shredding the documents in the office. Do not try to dispose of these papers in your home trash. Unfortunately, there are dishonest individuals who search trash cans looking for credit receipts or other personal information. One day an agency employee noticed a familiar piece of paper floating around her alley. When she picked it up, she found that it was one of the agency forms containing client information. Fortunately, it was an agency employee who found the paper. The individual who disposed of the form probably thought that it had been handled properly.

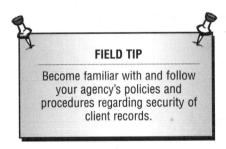

FIELD TIP

Become familiar with and follow your agency's policies and procedures regarding security of client records.

Confidential Client Discussions

Maintaining confidentiality is a challenge for all health care personnel but, because of the work environment, it is a greater challenge to maintain it in home health. You may have clients who live in a mobile home park or apartment building where the neighbors watch out for each other. It is not unusual for a neighbor to be aware that you are the home care employee seeing the client and ask you how the client is doing. If it is a facility for senior citizens, you may be caring for more than one client living in the neighborhood. If the client is feeling fine, you may be tempted to respond that the client is fine, but then how would you respond later if the client is not fine. Your best response would be to tactfully tell the inquirer that you cannot give out that information but encourage him/her to phone the client. Then it would give the client the opportunity to choose what information is or is not provided. Additionally, the client may welcome the thoughtful call.

Another place where you must be cautious is in an assisted living or adult care facility. In some of those facilities the clients may have their own apartments but eat meals together. They tend to keep in close touch with each other and probably know more about each other than you will ever know. No matter how well they know each other, you do not want to join in the conversations. It is each client's prerogative to decide what information she/he shares with others. If you are up front with inquirers and tell them that you cannot share information about a client, it will also assure them that you could be trusted not to reveal information about them if they should ever become your clients.

When providing information about the client to a family member, you must be sure that it is with the client's consent. It is best to have the client share any specific information. The client may, however, wish to have you explain certain aspects of their illness to a relative. There are other aspects that the client may not want shared except by him or herself. Make sure you understand to what limits you should divulge information.

Everyone knows that they should never discuss clients in a public area, even if the discussion is with someone that needs the information. There is too much of a risk that you will be overheard. A relative of a hospital client was taking the bus home from the hospital. She overheard two people, employees of the hospital, discussing a client. She was sure that they were discussing her husband, and she was very upset about the incident. Whether or not it was her husband being discussed, the damage was done.

One area where you need to take particular precautions about discussing clients is in the parking lot of your agency. When out in the open, you may think that there is no one who can hear you, but there could be someone sitting in a car who you cannot see but who can easily hear you. If you do see someone in the parking area who shares the care of the same client and you need to discuss his/her care, tell your fellow employee that you need to talk to him/her inside without mentioning the client's name.

Most agencies do not have many private areas in which to discuss clients. Any employees who overhear conversations about clients need to remember that they are also bound to maintain confidentiality about the clients. If there happen to be non-employees in the office, find an area away from them to discuss clients. When clients are discussed in case conferences or in-service sessions, everyone needs to remember that the information remains in the room. When presenting a client situation, take care of the amount of information that is shared. Don't share information about the client that may be interesting but is not relevant. During in-service presentations, it usually is not necessary to share client names if you are using a client example to clarify a point.

The size of the community in which you are practicing can present its own challenges in relation to confidentiality. If you work in a metropolitan area, you may think that you do not have to worry about someone recognizing you or the individual you are discussing. The bus incident, discussed earlier, occurred in a large metropolitan area. In a small community, you have to take extra precautions regarding confidentiality. Usually everyone knows everyone else and you never know who is related to whom.

In a small community, it may be difficult to avoid caring for a close friend or even a relative. It is best to turn the client care over to a coworker but that may not always be possible. If you must care for the client, inform him/her as to your role as the practitioner. Seek guidance from your clinical supervisor to help you maintain objectivity while providing care.

Caution must be exercised if you happen to see clients or their family members in a public place, such as a grocery store. Asking them about their condition could inadvertently cause disclosure of some confidential information. Even well-meaning condolences can result in a breach of clients' privacy.

When discussing clients, ask yourself if this individual needs to know this information. Likewise when you are engaged in a conversation with another employee, ask yourself if this information is something you should know. Our work is interesting; it is easy to get caught up in inappropriate conversations that may be breaching someone's privacy. We need to help each other by reminding colleagues that a conversation may not be appropriate.

The clinical supervisor and physician need to have detailed information about the clients for whom they are responsible. Other staff members who share care for the client also need information but in less detail. Because you are visiting the client in his/her home, you will become privy to some information about the client and family that has no relevance to the client's care. That information should not be shared with anyone. It could be something that does not seem very significant to you, but it could be important to the client. Clients trust you to be discrete when they allow you to come into their homes. You do not want to break that trust.

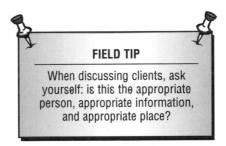

FIELD TIP

When discussing clients, ask yourself: is this the appropriate person, appropriate information, and appropriate place?

Technology

Modern technology creates new challenges for maintaining confidentiality. Caution needs to be exercised when leaving messages on answering machines. You never know who might listen to those messages. If you need to leave a message, do not use any client names or information; just let the individual know that you need to speak with him/her. The same precautions need to be observed when using a cellular phone. People can listen to conversations over cell phones. When you are at home, and are discussing a client on the phone, try to do it in a secure area. Instruct your family members that these conversations are confidential.

Home health employees should never give client phone numbers to any of their friends or family members. If they need to be able to reach you when you are at work, have them phone the agency office. The office staff will contact you with important messages. On the other hand, you should not give your phone number or address to clients. You may think that clients will not abuse the use of that information. Some clients have been known to waste time phoning the agency employee in an emergency. Give all clients a business card containing the office phone number. If they need to reach you, instruct them to phone the office and the agency staff will contact you. Assure them that you will return the call as soon as possible. Another advantage of providing a business card to all of your clients is that it helps them to remember your name when they want to reach you.

A new technology that sometimes creates problems is "Caller ID." Many times it is more convenient to phone clients from your home to verify appointments or when you are on-call. The problem is that with the "Caller ID" service, the client or family could identify your phone number. Modern phone systems have a code that you can enter before you dial the client's phone number in order to block the identification of your number. Some clients have phones programmed not to accept blocked numbers. If that is the situation with a client, the agency needs to notify him/her that the phone needs to be unblocked while the client is receiving services from the agency staff. Another option would be to phone that client from the office.

Home health agencies would probably not be able to function without a beeper system. During a visit, it is best to turn the beeper to vibrate, so if it goes off, it doesn't interrupt the client. This principle should be remembered when you are in a meeting too. Cell phones should also be turned off so they don't cause a distraction.

Confidentiality about Work Associates

Confidentiality responsibilities also apply to discussing our work associates, physicians, supervisors, administrators, and fellow employees. There are times when one or more of them may aggravate you but you must refrain from engaging in gossip about them. Sometimes the discussions may seem interesting, but you need to put yourself in their places and think about how you would feel. When engaging in these discussions, also consider whether the content could be considered slanderous.

CONFLICTS OF INTEREST

We must be aware of potential conflicts of interest that we may have in relation to our professional practice. You may not have any direct business connections that would constitute a conflict of interest but you may have a friend or relative who is associated with such a business, such as a durable medical equipment (DME) manufacturer or supplier. You need to declare any potential conflict that you have. Additionally you need to be cautious when making any recommendations to clients, e.g., when helping them choose a doctor or recommending where to purchase medical equipment. The best policy when making recommendations is to give at least three names. If you are associated with a health-related company on the list, you must also declare that information to the client.

As client advocates, we need to make clients aware of the importance of shopping around. There can be a great difference in costs between companies. Some items, such as shower benches, might be purchased more economically in a pharmacy or discount store than from a medical equipment company.

If your agency is associated with a company or health care provider that supplies a service that you have occasion to recommend, you must be cautious how you make the recommendation. You must provide a list of all providers of the service in that area and then indicate which one is associated with your agency.

CLIENT RIGHTS AND RESPONSIBILITIES

Client Rights

As client advocates, home health professionals must inform clients about their rights and ensure that those rights are protected. Table 9–1 contains a list of client rights. In addition to confidentiality, the clients have other privacy rights that must be ensured. When providing care in the home, it can be a challenge to provide privacy when needed. Occasionally, a bedbound client may be located in the front room of the home. You may have to help the nursing assistant determine how to ensure privacy during the bath.

Home care staff become proficient in improvising procedures to adapt to the environment. When you are new to home care, take advantage of the more seasoned home health professionals who have already encountered similar situations. Home care practitioners learn to adapt to a variety of situations, such as performing a dressing change for a client who lives in a car. Home health can pose many exciting challenges for the professional.

Table 9–1	CLIENT RIGHTS

Right to respect of self and property
Right to individualized care
Right to participate in planning care
Right to information about condition and treatment
Right to notification regarding financial responsibilities
Right to receive care without prejudice
Right to refuse care or portions of care
Right to information regarding resources
Right to protection of privacy and confidentiality privileges
Right to timely notice of discharge
Right to voice grievances about care
Right for guardian or family to exercise these rights when client is
   incapacitated

Be cautious about intruding on family time. Try to work around the family routines. This can be more of an issue when providing shift or respite care rather than with intermittent visits. Make sure that you allow family privacy for meals and when they are having a discussion. Make sure that the nursing assistants and nurses that you are supervising understand the importance of providing privacy for the entire family.

Clients have the right to participate in planning their care. In order to exercise this right, they need information about their condition and treatment. Teaching is a major responsibility of the home health professional. Clients also have the right to refuse treatment. You are responsible to make sure that clients understand the effects of their refusal, so that they are making an informed consent.

Clients are entitled to receive individualized care that meets their needs. Additionally they are entitled to participate in their discharge plan and be sufficiently informed about the intended date of discharge.

The home health professional is expected to advocate on behalf of the clients to coordinate their care. The coordination requires regular communication with the physician, agency staff, and other care providers. Home care practitioners need to provide sufficient information to third-party payors to ensure that the client receives approval for the required services. The practitioner must take care that visits are not wasted. Many insurance companies allow a limited number of visits per year for each client. If visits are used unnecessarily early in the year, and then the client requires more home care services later on, she/he may not be able to receive all of the needed services. Client advocacy also includes seeking out information about community resources that could benefit the client.

The clients have the right to know the name, title, and role of the individuals who are providing the services. This right is easier to facilitate in home health because each client tends to see a limited number of agency employees. In a structured facility, a client encounters several different employees and may become confused about the roles of the different staff members.

The clients are entitled to treatment with respect and without prejudice. Additionally, the care must be rendered regardless of how the agency is reimbursed. Likewise, clients have the right to expect respect for their property. In a structured facility, sometimes employees forget to ask permission before they open a drawer in the client's bedside stand or look in the client's closet. It is easier to remember not to open a closet or drawer in clients' homes. Make sure that you have clients' permission before handling their possessions. Avoid using the clients' supplies. This is one reason why home care personnel carry their own hand soap and towels.

Clients have the right to formulate advanced directives. These advanced directives can be in the form of a living will or durable (medical) power of attorney. A living will is intended to place limits on the extent of treatment to be administered. A durable or medical power of attorney appoints an individual to make health-care decisions on behalf of the client when she/he is unable to make those decisions. Additionally, even without a durable power of attorney, clients have the right to have family members or guardians exercise client rights in their behalf if they are unable to do so themselves. Copies of these advanced directives must be placed in the client's chart so they can be honored by everyone who cares for the client.

Finally clients have the right to voice grievances about their care without reprisal for doing so. It is expected that the agency will provide clients with names and telephone numbers of individuals to whom they can make their complaints. The Medicare COPs require that if there is a complaint, the agency will investigate the incident and document the complaint and its resolution.

Client Responsibilities

Along with rights, there are responsibilities. Just as clients are entitled to care regardless of age, race, color, national origin, religion, sex, or disability, they are also obliged to accept care from all health care staff without prejudice. Home health agencies try to accommodate clients' wishes but are not legally able to accommodate them if the wishes are based on prejudice.

While clients have the right to participate in planning their care, they also have the responsibility to provide accurate information about their condition and participate in learning about how to care for themselves. They are responsible to provide a safe environment for the agency staff to work. They are also responsible for storing their valuables in an appropriate place out of danger of damage or misplacement.

Clients need to notify the agency if they are not going to be available for a scheduled visit. Additionally, they need to inform agency personnel when they change their primary care physician or their third-party payor. Table 9–2 contains a list of client responsibilities.

PERSONAL INVOLVEMENT

There is greater risk for personal involvement with clients in home health than in other health care situations. This section discusses some of the pitfalls of personal involvement and how to avoid them.

Table 9–2	CLIENT RESPONSIBILITIES

The client is responsible to:
- Accept agency services without prejudice
- Participate in planning of care
- Provide accurate information about condition
- Participate in learning activities about treatment
- Accept responsibility for own health care
- Accept consequences for refusal of treatment
- Pay for services as agreed in service agreement
- Provide a safe environment for self and agency staff
- Keep valuables in secure area
- Notify agency when not available for a scheduled appointment
- Notify agency about change in physician or third-party payor

Home care practitioners tend to care for the client for a longer period of time than occurs in an acute care facility. Usually fewer staff members share the client's care than would be the case in a structured facility. Most clients are likable and appreciative of the fact that the staff come to provide care in their homes. Because of these factors, there is a greater chance for the clients to become attached to their agency caregivers and vice versa.

We need to remember these risks so we do not become too personally involved with our clients. We can help the clients more by maintaining a professional relationship. This includes avoidance of sharing personal information with clients and discussing personal problems. For example, it is probably not harmful for the client to be aware that you have a spouse and children but you would want to avoid providing detailed information, such as the place of your spouse's employment. It is never appropriate to bring any family members or pets to see the client; even if the client has indicated an interest in the family. You do not want to share problems you may be having with a family member.

The client may ask what you did over the weekend. A brief response would be appropriate, but then you should turn the conversation back to the client. It may be that the client initiated the conversation so she/he could discuss something that happened to him/her that weekend.

Home health practitioners need to learn to set professional boundaries when providing care. The difficulty with setting boundaries is that they are recognized more easily once they have been crossed. Recognition that the boundaries can be vague is a good first step toward establishing a therapeutic relationship. One can learn by experience, including from other home health personnels' experiences.

Setting boundaries can be accomplished by creating a professional environment. The focus of the relationship should always be on the client. This can be facilitated by educating the clients as to the practitioner's role. Clients also need to learn the practitioner's expectation of the client role. This education ideally begins when the client is admitted to agency services and the ground rules are established.

Begin preparing the client for the time when the therapeutic relationship is discontinued. At the time of discharge, goodbyes need to be said. The client needs to know who should be called if any problems arise. It needs to be clarified that any renewed contact will be through a contractual arrangement.

Be cautious if the client begins to compare you favorably to family members, for example, should the client indicate that you care for him/her better than a daughter or son. Although such a comparison may be flattering, it may also indicate a need to help the client establish better communication with the family member. You also need to be cautious that you are not instrumental in creating problems between the client and family members.

Take care that you do not get involved in discussions of sensitive topics. The general rules are not to discuss politics, religion, or any other controversial subjects. The client may initiate the subject. You can listen for a short time and then tactfully return the subject to why you are there: to provide skilled services. Avoid giving your opinion on family matters.

Another issue that frequently arises is the acceptance of gifts. This becomes an issue, especially, during the holiday times. Accepting gifts of money is never appropriate. Some clients think that they need to tip some staff members, such as nursing assistants or housekeepers. The clients need to be assured that their care has already been paid for fully. Accepting a purchased gift is also not appropriate. One type of gift that may occasionally be proper is a small home-made item, created by the client, as a memento. Even then, be cautious about accepting the gift. Some clients may give a gift as a means to manipulate the employee. If you feel that accepting the gift will affect your professional objectivity, do not accept the gift.

SPECIAL CIRCUMSTANCES

Non-compliant has become a highly used label for clients who have difficulty following their prescribed medical regimen. We must be cautious about placing this label on clients. When a client does not seem to follow their medical treatment regimen, you need to find out why. If the client is labeled as non-compliant, it releases everyone from the responsibility of solving the problem. Make sure that the client understands the importance of the treatment and the consequences if it is not followed. Be sure that there is not some other reason that prevents the client from being compliant. That issue may have to be resolved before the client is ready to deal with his/her own illness.

Frequently, home health personnel work for more than one agency or institution. If you do work for more than one facility, remember that you must maintain confidentiality between the facilities. In small communities, you may even take care of the same client at both facilities. Any information that is shared must come by way of the official routes. If you accept a case at one agency, you need to follow through on that commitment. If you receive a better offer from the other agency, it is not appropriate to renege on your original commitment.

Home health professionals are required to maintain the ethical standards of their profession. The basic premise is to "do no harm." It is beneficial for an agency to periodically take the time to have a general discussion of ethical issues with all levels of employees. As an individual practitioner, take advantage of discussions with your colleagues about various ethical situations.

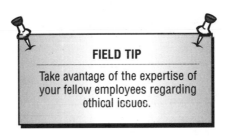

FIELD TIP

Take avantage of the expertise of your fellow employees regarding ethical issues.

References

Arizona Certified Agency Policy Manual: COP Interpretive Guidelines for Home Health Agencies, pp. B-14 to B-20. Phoenix, Department of Health Services, 1997.

Hilliard L. S.: Manager's Corner: Innovative or Disintegrate. Home Care Nurse News, 1998; 5(6):1, 2, 8.

Management and Evaluation of a Care Plan. The Beacon Homecare FOCUS Series, 1996; pp. 1–16.

Medicare Reimbursement of Therapy Services. The Beacon Homecare FOCUS Series, Mequon, WI, Beacon Health, 1996; pp. 1–9.

Neighbors, M. and Monahan, F. D.: A Practical Guide to Medical–Surgical Nursing in the Home, sections 1 and 6. Philadelphia, W.B. Saunders Co., 1998.

Olsten Health Services: Transitional Nurses Orientation Learner Guide, pp. 10–2 to 10–8. Melville, NY, Olsten Health Services, 1997.

Peterson, E., and Solomon, D.: Maintaining Healthy Boundaries in Professional Relationships: A Balancing Act. Home Care Provider, 1998; 3(6):314–318.

Salminen, C.: Designating Your Compliance Officer. AAHC Arizona Homefront, 1998:15(11):1.

Schmid, M. M. and Liaschenko J.: Ethical Issues in Infection Control in Home Care. Home Care Provider, 1999; 4(1):8–9.

Sperling, R.: How OASIS relates to the Medicare 485. Home Healthcare Nurse, 1999; 17(2):82–85.

Wellmark Fiscal Intermediary: Medicare Guide to Billing for HHAs, pp. 16–22. Des Moines, IA, Wellmark, Inc., 1997.

Legal Aspects

This chapter explores medical-legal issues as they relate to home health care. Legal issues relating to fraud and abuse, abandonment, antitrust concerns, and transporting clients are just a few aspects that are addressed.

CORPORATE COMPLIANCE

The law holds corporate officers responsible for ensuring that the company and employees follow federal and state regulations. If an employee is found to be harassing other employees or clients or an employee is committing fraud, not only will the employee be held responsible for his/her acts but the employers will also be held responsible. Hence, it behooves the employers to do everything possible to uphold the policies based on state and federal laws.

The Office of the Inspector General (OIG) of Health and Human Services recommends a compliance program guide for home health agencies to help meet this responsibility. The recommendations include the appointment of a compliance officer who will be responsible for developing a corporate code of conduct. An education program to educate employees about the compliance program and set up communication systems to monitor the program are recommended. Many agencies already have a corporate compliance program in place. Whether or not your agency has a formal program, you, as an employee, are responsible for being knowledgeable about the agency's policies regarding these laws.

The OIG guidelines for a corporate compliance program include the following ethical/legal issues:

Appointment of a compliance officer
Written policies (Code of Conduct) which include:
 Antitrust laws
 Confidentiality
 Conflicts of interest
 Copyright, trademark, and trade secrets
 Equal opportunities
 Immigration laws
 Sexual harassment
 Substance use and abuse
 Fraud and abuse
 Health, safety, and environmental issues
 Involvement with political process
 Discrimination
 Abandonment
 Advanced directives
 Creation of hot lines for employees to report suspected violations
 Development of procedures for employees who detect violations

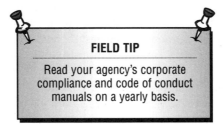

FIELD TIP

Read your agency's corporate compliance and code of conduct manuals on a yearly basis.

Antitrust Laws

Federal and state laws forbid a competitor to exercise unreasonable economic control over the marketplace.

Impairing competition through price fixing, illegal bidding, and kickbacks fall under these antitrust laws.

Kickback laws prohibit anyone from giving or receiving payment in exchange for referrals. Agencies need to be cautious when marketing their services. Leaving presents at hospitals, physician offices, or with clients could look suspiciously like kickbacks. Doing favors like running errands or providing extra services for the client could be considered an inducement for a referral. You also need to be cautious about accepting money or gifts from someone, such as a durable medical equipment (DME) company, who may want you to make a recommendation for the company's services. Both offering and receiving kickbacks are illegal.

The Balanced Budget Act of 1997 prohibits discrimination of referrals made for client services. If your agency is associated with another related business, e.g., a hospital, when making a recommendation to the client about the business, you must provide a list of other similar businesses in the service area and make the client aware which one is owned by the agency's company. If you or a relative happens to have a business interest in a company whose products or services you may have occasion to recommend, you must inform the client of other similar businesses in the area and make your relationship to the company known. You also must make your business interests known to your agency. These practices will help you avoid giving the impression of a conflict of interest.

Fraud and Abuse

Fraud and abuse in the health care industry are major concerns of the federal government and the general public. Unfortunately, the general perception is that the majority of home health agencies do abuse the Medicare system. Some of the changes that we are dealing with as a result of the Balanced Budget Act of 1997 were legislated in an effort to combat fraud and abuse.

In 1965, when the Medicare and Medicaid programs were created, Congress incorporated provisions to prevent fraud and abuse into the law. Over the years, these laws have been expanded. The Health and Human Services Office of the Inspector General is responsible for enforcing these provisions.

Fraud is defined as intentionally, knowingly, and willfully making false statements to obtain benefit or payment for non-qualifying services. False billing claims and misrepresenting services provided are examples of fraud.

Abuse is defined as unknowingly or unintentionally employing practices that directly or indirectly result in unnecessary costs to the Medicare program. The main difference between fraud and abuse is whether the act is intentional. Providing medically unnecessary services and charging greater amounts for services for Medicare clients than for non-Medicare clients are examples of possible abuse.

In 1995, the Health Care Financing Administration (HCFA) initiated Operation Restore Trust (ORT) to target Medicare fraud and abuse in health care, including the home health industry. The ORT surveyors investigate agency's records and policies looking for evidence of fraudulent billing practices. The targeted agencies are chosen based on a number of factors that raise suspicions, including excessive visits per client and inflated cost reports.

Some issues that an ORT surveyor will evaluate are:

Billing for
items or services not actually rendered
medically unnecessary services

      duplication of bills
      client not homebound
      inadequate or substandard care
      unqualified services
      unqualified or unlicensed personnel
      falsified visit notes or plans of care
      forged beneficiary signatures
      duplication of services
Failure to return overpayments
Incentives to actual or potential referral sources
Joint ventures between parties that can refer to each other
Improper client solicitation
Discriminatory admission and discharge of clients
Client abandonment

The ORT surveyors examine client records to make sure that the visit documentation supports the bills submitted for Medicare reimbursement. This is where the home health professional comes into the picture.

The list of improprieties that the surveyors are looking for should demonstrate how crucial documentation can be. There must be on-going and accurate documentation of the client's medical condition and homebound status. The various records documented by different staff members will be compared for consistency of the description of the client's status. There needs to be evidence that the plan of care is being followed by all staff members. Surveyors examine the visit notes to make sure that there is no duplication of services and that skilled services are rendered appropriately and by properly qualified staff members.

The OIG surveyors pay special attention when examining client records to verify that the services are medically necessary and that the client is actually homebound. The OIG reports that homebound status has become the major issue in denials for reimbursement and suspicion of abuse. Evidence that raises red flags regarding home-bound status is documentation that indicates the client is no longer homebound but that Medicare services continue to be provided. Another concern is if there is no evidence of on-going evaluation of the client's homebound status.

The best safeguard to avoid survey problems is to keep up to date with the Medicare regulations. The greatest challenge is developing a working knowledge of the conditions of participation (COP), but once this is achieved, do not think you can sit back and relax. There are continual changes in the COPs, their interpretations, and how they need to be implemented. Further, the home care professional is responsible to re-evaluate the client needs to ensure that appropriate services are being provided. The burden of ensuring that the services continue to be medically necessary is not totally the physician's. The home care agency is still responsible to evaluate the client for eligibility for services and keep the physician informed about the client's status.

The surveyor will compare records to make sure there is consistency between staff members on documentation of the mileage and travel time required to make the visit. Accuracy is especially important when recording visit notes. Exact times must be recorded for travel, the actual visit, and documentation. Rounding up numbers is not acceptable. If it takes you 3 1/2 minutes to drive to the client's home, do not round the travel time up to 5 minutes. Surveyors become suspicious if a given employee always takes 5, 10, or 15 minutes to travel. In like manner, the mileage needs to be recorded in terms of the actual odometer reading. Usually the last three digits of the odometer figure are sufficient.

Bills for visits cannot be submitted for reimbursement until the visit notes are in the office. Therefore, you need to make sure that your visit notes are submitted in a timely manner. You may not worry about when you are paid for a specific visit, but your delays could also delay reimbursement for the visits to the agency.

There is a limit set by each state by which time orders must be signed by the physician and returned to the agency. You are responsible for submitting any phone or verbal orders as soon as possible so they can be sent to the doctor for signature. Additionally, you do not want to vary from the plan of care without approval from the doctor. Finally, the agency cannot bill for services until the signed orders for those visits are on file in the office.

There may be an occasional mistake with documentation, such as forgetting to record homebound status. Surveyors are more likely to look for a pattern of inaccuracies and inconsistencies rather than isolated incidences. They have designated a certain percentage of inaccurate records as an indication of fraud. If strong evidence of fraud and abuse is found, the OIG is prepared to revoke the agency's license. On a lesser note, if records are found that do not support bills that have already been paid by Medicare and the agency is not able to produce the appropriate documentation, the money will have to be returned. If you follow the basic principles of accurate and complete documentation, you should not have to worry about causing problems for your agency.

As a supervisor of nursing assistants and Licensed Practical Nurses (LPNs), you are responsible for making sure that they are following the care plan for the client. If you find that the documentation does not reflect the plan, you need to call it to the attention of the CNA or LPN.

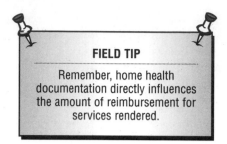

FIELD TIP

Remember, home health documentation directly influences the amount of reimbursement for services rendered.

A more serious offense is outright false documentation. An example of fraudulent documentation is when a nurse or therapist who is running behind on visits phones the client to determine how she/he is doing and then writes it up as though a visit had been made. The OIG surveyors will compare client signatures on the visit notes to look for forgeries.

Another fraudulent situation is when a home health professional omits information about the client's medical status or inaccurately describes the client's homebound status in order to continue providing services. If these practices are discovered, the agency and the personnel involved could be excluded from participation in Medicare or Medicaid programs. If the professional is included in the exclusion, that person would not be able to work in any health care institution that receives Medicare or Medicaid funds during the period of exclusion. This would cover most types of health care providers in the United States. Besides facing the threat of exclusion, individuals could be convicted of fraud. At the very least, the agency, if convicted, will have to pay restitution and possibly a fine.

Clients can be educated about how they can help prevent health care fraud and abuse. Measures that they can take include:

Obtaining and reading the benefit brochure from their third-party payor

Using health care providers with good reputations

Knowing the client rights and responsibilities

Verifying the identity of the health care provider before releasing insurance information

Reading forms thoroughly before signing

Obtaining billing information in writing

Taking an active part in planning their care

Refusing to accept unneeded services

Checking with their doctor if provided services or supplies not requested

Keeping a record of services and supplies provided

Reviewing statements sent by insurance companies.

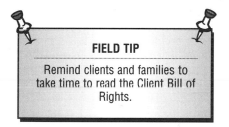

FIELD TIP

Remind clients and families to take time to read the Client Bill of Rights.

Abandonment

There is always a concern that medical providers will abandon the care of their clients if the reimbursement for the services becomes unprofitable. With the institution of a prospective payment system, HCFA is assuming that home health agencies will balance their mix of clients so that short-term clients will be in balance with the clients who require long-term care. Therefore, the agency will remain financially solvent. When Medicare reimbursement was paid per visit for as long as the services are reasonable and necessary, agencies did not become concerned about the clients who continued to require services over an extended period of time. But when a beneficiary cap is put in place, if a given client is admitted with a diagnosis of diabetes mellitus and later has a cerebrovascular accident (CVA), the agency staff needs to decide if they have the resources to continue the client's care. When terminating the client's services, there is always a risk of the agency being accused of abandonment.

Abandonment is defined as the unilateral termination of client services by the medical provider without reasonable notice and when further attention is required. There are three items that a client must demonstrate in order to prove abandonment. The three elements are:

The termination is unilateral
There was no reasonable notice
Further attention is needed.

If the client in some way played a part in the termination or agreed to it, the termination was not unilateral. If the client still needs care but payment from third-party payors is no longer available, the agency can offer the option of services on a private pay basis. If the client declines because she/he cannot afford the services, she/he has agreed to the termination. The offer and the client's response must be documented. It is recommended that a case conference be held to discuss the possible termination of the client before actually giving the client notice. The doctor also must be notified immediately in writing about the agency's intent.

Reasonable notice is the second element to be proved for abandonment. Some providers estimate that 30 days is required to provide reasonable notice. Some lawyers indicate that 3 to 5 days provides sufficient notice. State regulations and agency policy need to be considered when determining reasonable notice. The participants in the case conference can determine what would be reasonable notice for that particular client.

Notice is not required if the client no longer meets the eligibility requirements, such as if the client is no longer homebound. Violence or threats of violence by the client or a family member are grounds for immediate termination. Further, notice is not required when services are reduced instead of discontinued.

Notice must be in writing and delivered to the client's home. A discharge plan must be developed and implemented for the client who is terminated. If a discharge plan has been developed and discussed with the client at the time of admission, there should be little question of abandonment. The plan should include suggesting alternate sources of care for the client. When the date for termination of services arrives, the termination must be carried out.

The issue that no further attention is needed has to be considered. Whether further attention was needed is usually determined retrospectively. The court will examine if the client was injured as a result of the termination. Proof of physical injury or damage is usually required to demonstrate this element of abandonment. The agency needs to make every effort to ensure that the client's physical well-being is not jeopardized, including, if necessary, calling for an ambulance to transport the client to the hospital. If the client refuses the ambulance, she/he is contributing to the injury.

Caution needs to be exercised by the agency when working to control the case mix. It is far easier to control the mix at the time of admission. Medicare certified agencies are not allowed to discriminate against Medicare clients, however. If the agency declines to accept a Medicare client because of the severity of illness, then it cannot accept a non-Medicare client with a condition that has the same level of severity.

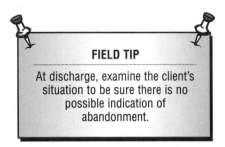

FIELD TIP

At discharge, examine the client's situation to be sure there is no possible indication of abandonment.

SPECIAL ISSUES

Any indication of discrimination needs to be avoided on the part of both the employer and employees. The Civil Rights Act of 1964 prohibits discrimination against employees because of race, color, religion, sex, or national origin. The Age Discrimination Act of 1967 prohibits the discrimination of employees 40 years or older, strictly because of their age. In 1990, the Americans with Disabilities Act was passed. HCFA requires equal access to health care without discrimination against clients by any health care provider participating in the Medicare program. Some specific types of clients protected under these laws are minors, the elderly, and clients with human immunodeficiency virus (HIV) infection or acquired immunodeficiency syndrome (AIDS), and disabilities.

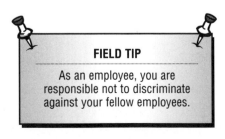

FIELD TIP

As an employee, you are responsible not to discriminate against your fellow employees.

Federal and state governments and the general public are becoming more concerned about the backgrounds of personnel caring for the sick and elderly. This is a legitimate concern, since individuals receiving the care are most vulnerable. Many home health agencies have been performing criminal background checks on potential employees for several years. In the last few years, states have been passing new legislation requiring criminal background checks on all employees who come in contact with clients in home health, extended care facilities, and adult care homes. Some agencies also require new employees to submit to drug screening. These agencies want to be assured that they are sending reliable personnel into clients' homes.

Clients have the legal right to view their own medical records. All agencies have policies regulating how this process is handled. It is not wise to allow the client to read the chart unsupervised, because there are many statements that could be misinterpreted by a reader who is unfamiliar with medical terminology.

Health care professionals are required to be knowledgeable about and follow their agency's policies and procedures. Agencies need to place all of their manuals with their policies, procedures, and governmental regulations in an accessible area for the employees. The employee can be liable if injury is caused because an agency policy was not followed.

Agency personnel are responsible for following the copyright laws. When preparing handouts for client teaching, make sure that you have permission to use any copyrighted materials from textbooks or professional journals.

CLIENT SIGNATURE

There are several forms, including visit notes, that usually require the clients signature. Unless someone else has a legal power of attorney, no one else can sign for the client. A medical power of attorney does not give another person the right to sign for the client. A medical or durable power of attorney indicates that a person has been designated to make health care choices for the client if she/he is incapacitated and unable to make the choices but not to sign legal documents.

There are occasions when the client is suddenly rendered incapable of signing his/her name, e.g., after a CVA. If the client still has the mental capacity to make decisions and can make a mark, have him/her do so and then have the spouse or family member sign to verify the client's mark. If the client no longer has the mental capacity to sign, have the family member sign and then document clearly why this was necessary. Advise the family to obtain the legal power of attorney as soon as possible.

TRANSPORTING CLIENTS

Follow your agency's policy regarding transporting clients. Some states designate, in the case of an accident, that the primary insurance used is the auto insurance covering the involved vehicle(s). In other words, if you are transporting a client in your car, your auto insurance will be the primary insurance to cover any damage or injuries.

The general rule is not to transport clients in your vehicle. There are always other options such as cabs or vehicles owned by the client's family or friends. Become knowledgeable about which cab companies or other agencies provide transportation for the disabled. If the client needs to get to the hospital rapidly, perhaps it would be better to summon an ambulance.

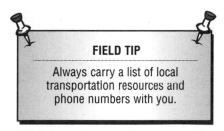

FIELD TIP

Always carry a list of local transportation resources and phone numbers with you.

There are occasions when it is part of the plan of care to transport the client somewhere such as to the doctor's office. Some agencies have the client sign a waiver to indicate that she/he understands that the agency's staff member will transport the client in the client's car and the client will be responsible in case of an accident.

PHYSICIAN ORDERS

Physicians need to be kept informed about their clients' progress. Communicating with physicians in home health is more challenging than it is in a structured facility. In structured facilities, the professional has the opportunity to speak with the doctor face to face. That rarely occurs in home health. It is even a challenge to speak directly with the physician over the phone because either you are out making visits or the doctor is unavailable.

Frequently, you need to communicate through one of the doctor's office personnel. It is crucial to document all communications, even those with unsuccessful outcomes. Include the name of the individual with whom you spoke. If you are unsuccessful in obtaining a needed order because the physician fails to return your call, you must persist. Merely charting that you received no response does not release you from your responsibility to the client. Keep the clinical supervisor informed of any physician communication problems. The supervisor may be able to make a helpful suggestion or intervene for you.

If you receive a negative response from a doctor, remind him/her that the response will be documented. Often this will encourage the physician to be more responsive to the clients' needs.

Some physicians respond better by means of a fax, whereas others prefer the phone. It is helpful if the agency keeps an updated file or book with the preferences of each doctor. The doctors will probably be more responsive if staff members consistently follow those preferences. Keep in mind how frustrating it must be for physicians to receive communications from several different staff members and have to explain their preferences to each one. Whether communicating with the physician via phone or fax, it is helpful to be specific about the response you are anticipating.

CONSUMER FRAUD

Many home health clients are prone to be subject to consumer fraud. The best prevention is to educate the client to be wary of different scams. Sometimes the home care employee becomes aware that the client is being taken advantage of by scam artists. The promotion of medical products, such as durable medical equipment or types of unproven treatments are examples of potential scams.

Consumer fraud is defined as a situation when a seller makes false promises to sell a product by misrepresentation of the product or its cost. The product may cost three to four times more than the cost of buying it in a store. Cost alone is not an example of fraud; however, a deceptive sales promotion could constitute fraud. Different types of scams that may possibly be considered as fraud are contests, telemarketing, home repair promotions, pyramids, and elaborate funeral home services.

Some red alerts to observe for include:

A push to make a quick decision

A request for the client's credit card number

A company whose only address is a Post Office Box number

An offer that supposedly has no strings attached

A requirement to phone a "900" or "809" (outside US) telephone number to receive a prize

A requirement to provide a good faith donation to receive a prize

If a home improvement scam:

    The contractor's car has an out-of-state license

    The contractor cannot provide references

    The contractor wants to be paid in cash only

If it looks too good to be true, it probably is.

Most state attorney general offices encourage citizens to report possible instances of consumer fraud. That governmental office is also a good resource if you or the client has questions about a potential scam.

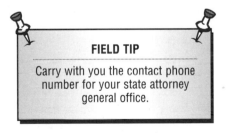

FIELD TIP

Carry with you the contact phone number for your state attorney general office.

INCIDENT REPORTS

As in a structured facility, incidents must be recorded in the case of injury or potential injury to the client or his/her property. Many agencies will initiate incident reports even if an agency staff member was not present at the time of the incident. For example, if the client informs a staff member that she/he fell, it is important to make a record of the accident. Later, if there is suspicion of client abuse because of bruises, these records will help provide background data for the investigators. When abuse is investigated, anyone having direct involvement with the client will be included in the investigation, including agency staff. If the client has frequent falls, the agency case manager may have to assess whether the home is a safe place for the client.

There is an increased risk of damage to the client's property in the home. The agency employee could accidentally break a lamp or vase in the home. Of course, we need to take precautions that we do not damage anything that belongs to the client. But if damage does occur, an incident report is needed. The agency is responsible for reimbursing the client for the loss. If you cause damage to the client's property with your car, your auto insurance will probably be considered the primary insurance. The best way to avoid causing damage with the car is to avoid driving onto the property. If you cannot avoid parking on the property, take extra precautions so that you do not run into a fence or cause some other damage.

PREVENTION

Prevention is always the most effective means to deal with the legal aspects of client care. Probably the most effective means of prevention is through open communication with the client and family. If we treat the client with respect and take responsibility for our actions, the client is less likely to want to initiate legal action against us. Of course, open communication will not help if we are careless about following agency policies and procedures, including thorough documentation.

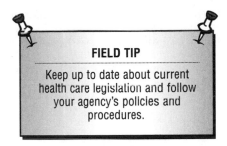

FIELD TIP

Keep up to date about current health care legislation and follow your agency's policies and procedures.

Home health professionals can avoid legal problems only by remaining well informed of the legal aspects that affect their practice. Pleading ignorance of the law is not a defense. As professionals, we are responsible for knowing and following current laws governing home health practice.

References

Arizona Certified Agency Policy Manuel: COP Interpretive Guidelines for Home Health Agencies, pp. B–13 to B–20. Phoenix, Department of Health Services, 1997.

Avoiding Fraud and Abuse Charges. The Beacon Homecare FOCUS Series, 1996; Medicare Reimbursement for Therapy Services, Mequon, WI, Beacon Health, 1996, pp. 15–16.

Calfee, B.: Labor Laws Working to Protect You. Nursing 96; 26(2): 34–39.

Fraud and Abuse in the Home Health Services Field. AHA Legal Alert, pp. 1–3. Washington D.C., American Hospital Association, 1997.

Health Care Financing Administration: Home Health Agency Manual (HIM-11) Chapter I, General Information about the Program, Sec 100, pp. 6–8. Washington, D.C., Department of Health and Human Services, 1992.

Hogue, E.: Avoiding Liability for Abandonment in an Environment of Reduced Medicare Utilization. Arizona Homefront, 1998; 15(3): 5–7.

Hogue, E.: Avoiding Liability for Termination of Services/Abandonment (Handout). Burtonsville, MD, 1998.

Hogue, E. E.: Communications with Physicians (Handout). Burtonsville, MD, 1998.

Hogue, E.: HCFA Addresses Issues Related to Termination of Services. Arizona Homefront, 1998; 15(9):6–7.

Hogue, E.: How to Deal with Today's Challenges of Managing Patient Mix. Arizona Homefront, 1999; 16(2):6.

Home Health Compliance Risk Areas as Identified by the OIG. Home Care Compliance Alert, 1998; 2(9).

Law Watch: A Legal Newsletter. Chicago, Foley Lardner Weissburg & Aronson, 1998.

Medicare Bulletin #416, by bcc (Blue Cross Calif) Fiscal Intermediary, Oxnard, CA, July 13, 1998, p. 13.

Medicare Bulletin #414, by bbc (Blue Cross Calif) Fiscal Intermediary, Oxnard, CA, March 25, 1998, p. 12.

Medicare Fraud and Abuse: Understanding the Law. Johnson, J. (ed)., Introduction. Washington D.C., National Health Lawyers Association, 1986.

Neighbors, M. and Monahan, F. D.: A Practical Guide to Medical-Surgical Nursing in the Home, Sections 1 & 6. Philadelphia, W. B. Saunders Co., 1998.

Salminen, C.: (Yet another) Corporate Compliance Update. AAHC Arizona Homefront, 1998;15(10):5.

Salminen, C. Designating Your Compliance Officer. AAHC Arizona Homefront, 1998;15(11):1.

Setting the Record Straight: An Industry Response to Fraud and Abuse. Homecare, pp. 19–20. Washington D.C., National Association for Home Care, 1998.

Stoker, J.: Congress's Report Card on Home Care Progress. Home Healthcare Nurse, 1999; 17(3):158.

Weissenstein, E.: Home Health 'Guidelines' include Mandates. Modern Healthcare, 1998; Aug:6.

Wellmark Fiscal Intermediary: Medicare Guide to Billing for HHAs, p. 15. Des Moines, IA, Wellmark, Inc., 1997.

Woods, G.: Telephone Scams and Older Consumers (brochure). Phoenix, Arizona Office of the Attorney General, 1995.

Special Issues

T his chapter discusses other special circumstances that affect the home health professional, including shift work, respite care, and professional appearance.

SHIFT WORK

A growing aspect of service from home health agencies is the provision of shift care. Shift care may involve the provision of private duty or respite services anywhere from 2 hours at a time to around the clock. During recent years, third-party payors have recognized the value of providing support for families to care for clients at home rather than admitting them to acute or long-term care facilities. Additionally, some families find that paying for private duty services for their family member is more cost effective and provides more comfort than care in a skilled nursing facility. Some home health agencies have learned to balance the client mix between intermittent care that is reimbursed by Medicare or insurance and shift care. Those agencies have been able to maintain fiscal solvency better than the agencies that specialize in one or the other type of services.

Medicare generally reimburses for intermittent or part-time visits only, but some Medicaid programs provide for limited private duty or respite care. The Balanced Budget Act of 1997 provided a clarification of the coverage requirement for part-time or intermittent nursing and home health aide services. This clarification took effect on October 1, 1997. The clarification states that "part-time or intermittent home health aide and skilled nursing services" means that the services are furnished any number of days per week as long as:

> The combined skilled nursing and home health aide visits last less than 8 hours each day
> The visits last less than 28 hours per week
> There are some special cases that may qualify for up to 35 hours per week of services based on a review of each case.

These hours are not sufficient for some clients either because they require more hours per week or they require services for an extended period of time. Besides Medicaid, there are other payors that may be able to assist.

RESPITE CARE

Respite, which means a short interval of rest or reprieve, has become a popular concept for care in recent decades. Respite services have provided opportunities for families to take on the care of elderly and disabled family members without completely exhausting the family resources. Most states have recognized that a developmentally disabled child thrives more at home than in an institution. Other situations in which families could benefit from respite care are for clients with terminal illnesses or a progressively deteriorating condition, such as Parkinson's disease, multiple sclerosis, or Alzheimer's disease.

Generally, states will prioritize which clients will receive Medicaid-supported services. Clients who are victims of abuse, neglect or exploitation receive the highest priority. Other factors that are considered are:

> Availability of family resources
> Availability of community resources

Financial resources
Nature and severity of client's illness or disability
Need for 24-hour care by a family member
Family caregiver having difficulty coping
Mental status of client.

DISCIPLINES INVOLVED IN SHIFT WORK

The registered nurse or therapist is not as likely to be the one providing the care, but most likely will be supervising the agency staff member who does provide the care. There are some occasions, however, when the registered nurse does provide shift care. There are some agencies that provide private duty or respite care services for clients who are on ventilators or who are severely disabled. These clients will usually require the skills of a registered nurse (RN) or a licensed practical nurse (LPN). Another type of client who may require skilled nursing is the severely developmentally disabled child, especially one that requires oral or tracheal suctioning. Families with infants who require apnea monitoring may benefit from respite or private duty services. Without the assistance to the families through respite care, many of these clients would have to be institutionalized.

The majority of shift care cases are serviced by nursing assistants. There are many clients who benefit from extended nursing assistant services; for example clients with Alzheimer's disease or another type of dementia. Clients with a chronic illness, such as Parkinson's disease or chronic obstructive pulmonary disease, or with a terminal illness such as cancer may also benefit from these services. The number of hours of service provided to the client depends on the third-party payor source.

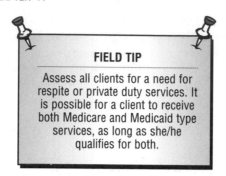

FIELD TIP

Assess all clients for a need for respite or private duty services. It is possible for a client to receive both Medicare and Medicaid type services, as long as she/he qualifies for both.

Another category of employee that may be used to provide private duty care, depending on the client's needs, is an attendant. State laws vary about the role of the attendant and if his/her use is allowed within the state. The state law will specify the extent of care that the attendant is allowed to provide. Usually attendant care is limited to assisting a client who requires supervision but is still able to participate in his/her activities of daily living with assistance.

These services may be a supplement to Medicare home health skilled nursing or therapy services. The private duty care may be coupled with other skilled services being reimbursed by a third-party payor. The requirements regulating these services will vary according to the third-party payor. The home care professional will need to become knowledgeable about those regulations that affect the client's care. If the client is receiving services reimbursed by both Medicare and another third-party payor, the practitioner needs to take care that the appropriate payor code is used for each visit note.

The discipline of the supervising professional will depend on the needs of the client and the plan of care. In some situations, supervising responsibilities may be shared by more than one professional. For example, a registered nurse may need to supervise the nursing assistant providing personal care while the physical therapist or occupational therapist is supervising the provision of range of motion exercises, ambulation, or activities of daily living.

CARE PLAN SUPERVISION

As discussed in Chapter 8, Case Manager Responsibilities, the care plan developed to guide the nursing assistant must be clearly written specifically for the client. The frequency of supervisory visits will vary according to the payor. The payor may require more frequent supervisory visits at the start of care and then less frequent ones as the care progresses.

Because of the number of hours that the staff member is present in the home, it is important to provide opportunities for the client and family to give input about who will be involved in the care. This input can be initiated when the client is being admitted to the agency services. The home health professional should encourage the client and family to participate in developing the care plan. Supervisory visits also provide another time for this input. Meeting the certified nursing assistant (CNA) at the client's home at the time of the assistant's first visit to orient the aide is always helpful. Providing orientation each time a new nursing assistant is used is not practical but, if orientation is provided with the most frequently used aides, future problems could be prevented. When there is a change in the agency caregiver, it would be helpful if the current aide meets the new aide at the client's home to provide an introduction and brief orientation.

Working the Night Shift

Some clients require private duty services during the nighttime. No matter which discipline is providing the services, the individual needs to realize that working shifts in the client's home, especially the night shift, is very different than in a structured facility. In an acute or long-term care facility, there are many clients and other staff to keep you stimulated. In the home there is one client and, it is hoped, she/he is able to sleep most of the night. If the home care employee just sits and watches the client, she/he very likely will fall asleep too. The family or third-party payor is paying a great deal of money to provide services to assist the client. Paying for someone to sleep is unacceptable.

The staff member needs to engage in quiet activities that will keep him/her mentally stimulated while the client is asleep. First, the client must be checked at least every hour to make sure she/he is still asleep and does not need assistance. The care plan may call for care to be rendered on a regular basis, such as changing the client's position or taking vital signs. The care plan for the CNA may call for some light housekeeping that can be done without waking the client.

The employee needs to bring some mind stimulating activities with him/her to fill the time when the care plan activities are completed. Each individual staff member knows what activities would be best for him/her. Some people find a good book to be stimulating whereas others would be asleep after the first few pages. Watching television has varying effects on people too. Other stimulating activities that might be used are some type of needlework or crossword puzzles. The home care employee needs to keep in mind that these activities are secondary to the client's care.

A nourishing meal also helps to stimulate energy in the employee during the shift. It is not appropriate to eat the client's food. Many clients are living on fixed incomes and cannot afford to feed the home care staff. The employee can bring a lunch and leave it in the client's refrigerator until it is needed.

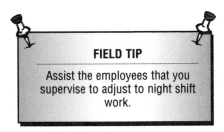

FIELD TIP

Assist the employees that you supervise to adjust to night shift work.

CLIENT/FAMILY SUPPORT

Home health private duty services provide an opportunity for the client to receive care without leaving home. Although this situation is preferred over care in a structured facility, the agency staff need to keep in mind that the presence of a person who is not a family member creates extra stress on the client and family. Agency employees need to work to alleviate that stress. The more control that the client and family feel they have over the situation the more easily they can cope.

It is a challenge for the home care employee who is providing private duty services to judge when the client and family members require some privacy. When providing care to the same client for an extended period of time, one may forget that the family members still need some time to themselves.

Mealtime may be one of those occasions. If the client is eating a meal with the family, the agency caregiver could take his/her lunch into another room. This also may provide a break for the employee. If there are no family members present to eat with the client, it may be therapeutic for the employee to eat his/her lunch at the same time to keep the client company. That judgment will have to be made according to the needs and wishes of the client.

ACTIVITIES FOR THE CLIENT

The care plan for the client receiving shift care should include activities that provide mental and physical stimulation, based on the client's mental and physical abilities. The basic rule is to provide one mentally and one physically stimulating activity per day.

The mental activities would need to be based on the client's cognitive ability and interests. An elderly or terminally ill client can be prompted to reminisce about good times by spending time viewing photo albums or family videotapes. Other mental activities that could be considered are watching a movie, reading a book, playing a board game, or working a jigsaw puzzle. If the client has dementia, a six-piece puzzle would be stimulating for him/her but not too difficult. Television is an acceptable activity, but is not recommended because the viewer is passive.

There are many physical activities that can be adapted to the client's physical ability. Exercise to music can be adapted to the client whether she/he is able to ambulate or not. The client who can ambulate even with an appliance, e.g., a walker, can still move around to the music. The bedbound client might still be able to move his/her arms and legs or at least move hands and feet to the music. Even this small amount of exercise can be beneficial to the client.

Other physical exercises that can be used include gardening, baking cookies, short walks, shopping if the client is not homebound, or making popcorn to eat while watching a movie. Gardening can be modified by planting a flower in a flower pot. An activity that can be both mentally and physically stimulating for the client with dementia is having him/her set the table and name the utensils as they are handled.

PROFESSIONAL APPEARANCE

Some agencies require that the home health staff wear uniforms or laboratory coats. Other agencies allow staff members to wear street clothing. This section focuses on what would constitute appropriate personal appearance for home health staff. Not only do home health professionals need to be concerned about their own appearance but they are responsible for noting the appearance of the staff that they supervise.

The highest standards of service and image are required of individuals working in the home care profession. They represent the agency. The following basic guidelines should be considered when selecting appropriate clothing and accessories. The employee's

Appearance should not be offensive to the client or family

Clothes should consist of garments that are practical for providing care (e.g., allow ease of movement and are easily cleaned)

Clothes and accessories must be designed to maintain medical asepsis

Most agencies probably have some type of dress code to provide guidance for the employees. Whether there is a dress code or not, many home health employees prefer to wear scrubs because they are easy to wash and are comfortable.

A good guideline on which to base your selection of attire is choose clothing that would appear appropriate to the majority of clients and families. Many home health clients are elderly and may have a more conservative view of appropriate appearance than younger clients. Always try to dress so you do not offend the client and family. Wear clothes that fit you, no matter what your size or body type. Shorts or short skirts may not be appropriate. Some clothing may be appropriate when relaxing at home but not when you are working.

It is best to avoid wearing clothing that contains logos or messages that could be offensive. Think about if this item is something that you would wear if you were working in a hospital or a skilled nursing facility. Since you cannot always predict whether a message or logo might be offensive, the best rule is to avoid wearing such clothing.

Jewelry is something that also needs to be considered. You may have some nice, expensive-looking jewelry that you like to wear. Consider how the jewelry will appear to a client who may not have sufficient money to pay for his/her medications. You also have to consider safety and medical asepsis issues when selecting jewelry. Expensive-looking jewelry may attract the attention of a dishonest individual. An elaborate ring could harbor microorganisms or even inadvertently scratch a client.

Another issue to consider is fingernails and nail polish. Designer nails may look very nice, but they may not be free of microorganisms. The color of the polish or the length of the nails may be offensive to the client. The client might be injured because of the nails' length.

Cologne or perfume also needs to be considered. Some dress codes suggest wearing a light fragrance. Some clients are allergic to fragrances and many home health clients have chronic lung conditions, so wearing no fragrance at all would be a better policy. Many clients will tell you that they experience difficulty breathing if there is someone who is wearing perfume nearby, even if that person is sitting clear across the room from them. Some clients may not feel comfortable telling the agency's employee that his/her fragrance is bothering them. We need to anticipate that this would be a problem for the client without him/her having to tell us.

Smoking is another issue. Smokers lose their sense of smell and do not realize how strong the odor of stale smoke can be on their clothing or in their hair. The smell could be particularly offensive to the client who feels nauseous.

The clothing needs to be practical in that you are able to perform your duties without being restricted. Washable clothing is a must to maintain medical asepsis. Shoes should be of a closed-toe style to protect the feet. Just like the client needs to wear supportive footwear, you need to do the same thing if you are going to be assisting the client.

Many times health care employees forget that they are role models for clients and family caregivers. If you preach that clients should wear protective shoes or always wash their hands but you don't, guess how seriously the client and caregiver will take your teaching?

If home care employees keep in mind that they are representing the agency and may be the only agency representative that comes in contact with that particular client and family, they should have an easier time remembering to maintain a professional appearance. Lastly, picture identification is always required. The client and family members need the assurance that they are always admitting an authorized agency employee to their homes.

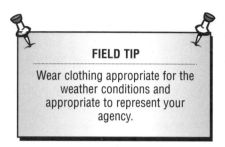

FIELD TIP

Wear clothing appropriate for the weather conditions and appropriate to represent your agency.

References

Dixon, B. T.: Help Patients Make Their Homes User-Friendly. Private Duty Homecare, 1998; Jan 13–14.

Dreyer, C. J.: Home Health Aide Supervision: Care Plans and Supervisory Visits. Home Health FOCUS, 1998; 5(6):45.

National Association for Home Care: HIM-11 Coverage Guide for Field Staff, 1998. Washington, D.C., National Association for Home Care.

Nissenboim, S. and Vroman, C.: The Positive Interactions: Programs of Activities for People with Alzheimer's Disease, 1998. Baltimore, Health Professions Press.

Schall, M. B. and Faria, S. H.: Intervention Strategies to Alleviate Family Stressors. Home Care Provider, 1997; 2(6):315–318.

Top 'dos and don'ts' of private duty home care: Eli's Home Health line, 1999; March 29:10–11.

Death in the Home

T he home care professional does not often need to deal with death in the home, but it is sometimes necessary. This chapter discusses the role of the home health nurse or therapist when caring for the client who is dying. The discussion will include options available to the dying client and family and when a hospice referral is appropriate.

RIGHT TO DIE AT HOME

The client's option to choose to die at home has become more of a reality with the growth of the home health and hospice industries. In most cases, the client can be more comfortable and gain more dignity when cared for at home. Home care provides a greater opportunity for the client's closer interaction with family and friends than is possible in the sterile hospital situation. The home situation especially provides for opportunities for the client to continue to have contact with his/her children or grandchildren and pets.

RIGHT TO ASSISTANCE IN ACCEPTING DEATH

Dr. Elizabeth Kubler-Ross was one of the first health care professionals to publicly deal with the dying client. She tells about the reception she received when she first began her research. When she searched a large general hospital, to identify some dying clients to interview, she found that no one on the entire hospital staff recognized that there were any dying clients in the hospital. After she found some clients who did recognize that they were dying, Dr. Kubler-Ross concluded that hospital staff tended to deny that any of their clients were dying.

Dr. Kubler-Ross was the theorist who first identified the five emotional stages of dying, which we still recognize today. Those five stages are denial, anger, bargaining, depression, and acceptance. Not only do the client and family experience these five stages when faced with death, but health care professionals also often experience these stages with each client for whom they provide care. Dr. Kubler-Ross was concerned that the health care professionals tended to lag behind the client in their acceptance of the client's death. This could create problems for the clients if those caring for them are not willing to recognize that they are dying and provide the badly needed comfort for their last days. Health care professionals have progressed a great deal from the days when Dr. Kubler-Ross first started her research; however, we need to continue to grow in our understanding of the needs of the dying client.

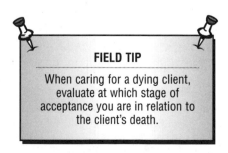

FIELD TIP

When caring for a dying client, evaluate at which stage of acceptance you are in relation to the client's death.

RIGHT TO CHOOSE EXTENT OF CARE

The client's plan of care needs to consider any advanced directives that the client may have written. The agency must have a copy of the advanced directive in order to honor the client's wishes. Regulations regarding advanced directives vary from state to state. You need to become familiar with the regulations within the state in which you practice. You also need to be familiar with your agency's policies regarding advanced directives.

Just because the client has a living will or knows that she/he is dying does not mean she/he does not want to be resuscitated. The client may not be ready to relinquish the right to decide about being resuscitated, and she/he may never get to that point. Some clients and families are more comfortable passing that control on to the individual who has the Medical Power of Attorney. Keep in mind that an advanced directive may be revoked at any time. This can be done verbally or in writing by the client, the physician, or the individual with legal responsibility.

It is important to discuss thoroughly with the client and family their wishes and to share that information with all of the staff members involved in the care of the client. Do not forget to include the nursing assistant in the loop of information. The aide is the one that tends to spend more time at the home than any other staff member. The aide may be the individual who will initiate care if the client has a sudden change in condition. Some home health professionals forget to keep in touch with or do not value input from certified nursing assistants (CNAs).

Frequently the client and family members share important information with the CNA. Unless specifically encouraged to do so, the nursing assistant may not share this information because she/he does not realize its significance. A wise home care professional would include the CNA in case conferences concerning the client.

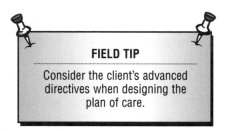

FIELD TIP

Consider the client's advanced directives when designing the plan of care.

RIGHT TO EXPRESS FEELINGS

Dr. Kubler-Ross noted that many dying clients experienced a sense of isolation from family, friends, and health care providers. It is to be hoped that we have improved from the time when she began her research. Some health professionals feel that they do not know what to say to a dying client. The client would respond that you do not have to say anything; just listen.

We recognize that an important task for the elderly in their later years is reminiscence. This also holds true for dying clients. Reminiscence assists individuals to validate their lives. By listening to the client's stories, you may be providing the most important part of the client's care. Teach family members and nursing assistants the importance of listening to these anecdotes. Encourage clients to share their stories. Photo albums and family videos facilitate reminiscence. A side benefit for the family is the perpetuation of the family history. For health care personnel, the stories can be interesting and you can gain a personal view of historical events.

RIGHT TO FREEDOM FROM PAIN

A major goal for the dying client's plan of care is to optimize the comfort and dignity of the client. This can be accomplished through treatment of primary and secondary symptoms such as pain, diarrhea, nausea, and vomiting. Additionally, the psychosocial and spiritual concerns of the client and family need to be acknowledged.

Pain management is a major concern that should be addressed in the plan of care. Pain can be a major fear for the dying client. Clients who are assisted to learn to manage their pain relief for themselves feel more relaxed and in control. Pain management should not only relieve pain but also maintain quality of life so the client is able to function as normally as possible.

Pain management begins with assessment of the client's pain. A thorough pain assessment needs to include all of the following elements:

Location of the pain and where it radiates
Pain intensity (e.g., 1–10 pain scale)
Client's description of pain: when it began; how long it persists; whether it is constant or intermittent
What makes the pain better
What aggravates the pain
How effective are medications and other interventions
How does pain affect sleep, mood, appetite, activities, and relationships
Other symptoms that accompany pain (nausea, sweating, dizziness, anxiety)
Meaning of the pain for the client
Coping mechanisms used by client
Client's attitude regarding use of pain medications
Cause of pain
Client's expectation regarding pain management.

In most situations, the client's pain can be controlled with a combination of pharmacologic and non-pharmacologic interventions. Frequently, pain is under-treated because of the unfounded fear of client addiction on the part of the health care professional, the client, or family members.

A three-step analgesic regimen developed by the World Health Organization provides useful guidelines for an effective pain management program. **Step 1** calls for the use of non-steroidal anti-inflammatory drugs, such as acetaminophen, for mild to moderate pain. In **Step 2,** an opioid analgesic is introduced when the pain persists or increases. Opioid drugs are effective to manage mild to severe pain. If the pain continues to increase and persist, management moves to **Step-3,** and the potency and dosage of the opioid are increased. The goal of pain management is to administer the appropriate dosage and frequency of analgesic medication needed to control the pain with the fewest side effects.

The following principles should be used when planning a pain management regimen.

Provide pain relief while allowing for an optimal level of functioning

Base plan on the pain assessment, including its etiology

Administer medication as easily as possible

Give pain medications orally whenever possible

Administer analgesics around the clock, not PRN

Medication for breakthrough pain is used PRN

Observe and treat side effects

Give the client and caregiver both oral and written instruction

Evaluate pain management program frequently and make changes as needed.

The client and family need to be educated about the pain management regimen. The learning process can be enhanced with handouts about the pain management plan and information about the medications, including expected side effects and measures to prevent or minimize side effects. The client and family need assurance that the requirement for higher doses of opioids does not indicate increased tolerance to the drug but instead indicates increased pain. Therefore, there is no need to be concerned when increasing the analgesic dosage.

Today, opioid analgesics are available in long- and short-acting forms. They can be administered orally, rectally, and transdermally, which provides increased client-control of pain management. Even when intravenous (IV) administration becomes necessary, portable IV pumps are available that can be controlled by the client. Pumps also help the client maintain mobility.

Effective pain management requires round-the-clock narcotic administration with the use of PRN medication for breakthrough pain. Adjunct analgesics, such as an antidepressant or antianxiety drugs, may prove useful to enhance the effectiveness of analgesics for some types of pain.

The client and caregiver should be encouraged to employ non-pharmacologic measures to enhance pain relief. The effectiveness of these measures will depend on the client's view of their value in relieving pain and promoting comfort. Heat will promote relief of aches and discomfort. Teach the client and caregiver to avoid burns by wrapping the hot pack in a towel. A cold pack may be preferred instead of heat and is used for 15-minute periods at a time. Massages are excellent to promote relaxation, stress relief, and distraction. Exercise is essential to mobilize stiff joints and strengthen weak muscles. When the client is incapacitated, range of motion exercises and repositioning will help relieve discomfort and prevent contractures and pressure ulcers. Immobilization of a body part is sometimes required to manage acute pain, but immobilization should not be used for prolonged periods of time.

Cognitive–behavioral interventions help the client develop a sense of control to cope with the pain. Encourage the client to try several modalities and decide which ones are most effective for him/her. Relaxation and imagery are effective for brief episodes of pain. Focusing attention away from pain or its side effects through prayer, music, talking, or exercise can be effective. A quiet, calm environment always contributes to the pain control regimen.

A thorough pain assessment needs to be made at least weekly to provide a basis for evaluation of the plan. Any report of increasing pain calls for additional assessments. When there is a change in the dosage or frequency of administration of the opioid analgesic, follow-up contact needs to be make the next day, at least by phone. It is also helpful if the client can keep a written log of the pain episodes, including the intensity of the pain and the effectiveness of the interventions.

RIGHT TO COMFORT

The client is assessed for other symptoms that may be caused by the pain medications or by the client's disease process. The home care professional needs to anticipate these symptoms and prevent them as much as possible.

Constipation

There can be many causes of constipation, including chronic opioid administration. If the client is undergoing a pain management plan, you should anticipate this side effect and work to prevent it or at least intervene early.

Keep in mind the three factors that promote bowel evacuation are exercise, fluids, and bulk in the diet. If the client's activity is limited, have the client compensate by increasing fluids. Most clients can find relief from constipation through the regular use of stool softners and a mild laxative used when needed.

Nausea and Vomiting

Antiemetics, such as thiethylperazine or diphenhydramine are usually effective against nausea and vomiting. If these symptoms are related to the use of narcotic analgesics, the effects will usually decrease after a few days. The client may experience sedation and mental clouding when antiemetics are used in combination with analgesics, but most clients tend to develop a tolerance to these sedative effects. Some clients may need to have a reduction in their analgesic dosage.

Some conservative measures that can be used in conjunction with or without antiemetic medications are to

Avoid large meals
Drink liquids between rather than with meals
Eat and drink slowly
Avoid sweet, fried, or fatty foods
Suck ice cubes, mints, or tart candies
Avoid bothersome odors
Avoid lying down immediately after meals
Wear loose-fitting clothes
Breathe deeply and slowly with episodes of nausea
Use distraction and relaxation techniques.

Diarrhea

Antidiarrhea medications may be needed if diarrhea is persistent. Some other measures that can be used to minimize diarrhea include:

Eating small, frequent meals

Avoiding high-fiber foods

Avoiding coffee, tea, alcohol, and sweets

Avoiding greasy or highly spiced foods

Avoiding milk if it aggravates the diarrhea

Eating high-potassium foods to replenish potassium

Drinking plenty of mild, clear fluids

Letting carbonated drinks lose their fizz before drinking

Following a clear liquid diet for a few days.

Respiratory Depression

When clients are on pain management, their caregivers must be educated to observe the clients for signs of respiratory depression. They will tend to develop tolerance to the respiratory depressant effects of the drugs after a few days of use. The family caregiver needs to know how to recognize when the respiratory rate becomes too low and what action must be taken if this occurs.

Anorexia

Anorexia is a common problem in elderly and dying clients. Risk factors for anorexia come from many sources. Some factors might be easily controlled. Assessments need to examine medications, therapies, changes related to the aging of the client, and possible infections. Cachexia, a combination of anorexia and abnormal metabolism of nutrients, is a common condition of the dying cancer client. Improving the client's appetite and increasing the nutritional intake can be a challenge. The client and family should be instructed about the following guidelines to improve the client's intake:

Make the food appealing
>   Use herbs, onions, garlic, or lemon
>   Arrange on attractive dishes
>   Provide pleasant, soft music
>   Use colorful placemats or napkins
>   Use a combination of hot and cold foods
>   Provide varied textures and colors of food
>   Provide fresh fruits to add flavor to bland foods

Provide mouth care before each meal
Maintain adequate fluid intake
>   Substitute fruit juice for coffee and tea

Review medications for anorexic side effects
Provide small, frequent meals
Provide fluids between meals rather than with them
Use high-energy proteins for supplements
Maintain a pleasant atmosphere
Provide pleasant conversations during meals.

If the client lives alone, Meals-on-Wheels is an appropriate option. Consider the option of a nutritional assessment by a dietitian. If the client has difficulty swallowing, a speech therapy referral may be appropriate.

Decubitis Ulcers

If the client is bedbound, the family caregiver requires instructions on how to care for the client and prevent unnecessary complications. Decubitis ulcers are a major concern. Caregiver education is crucial in order to prevent skin breakdown and other complications of prolonged bedrest. Do not assume that the caregiver knows that the client requires frequent changes in position, constant care to provide clean dry skin, skin massages with lotion, and good nutrition to prevent decubiti.

Reduced Energy

Depending on the client's condition, she/he may need information about how to conserve energy. Simple measures such as sitting during activities such as brushing teeth or helping with meal preparation can help keep the client active without exhausting his/her energy. Rest periods between activities are helpful. For example, resting after bathing and before ambulating is advisable for the weakened client. A referral to an occupational therapist may be necessary to help the client and caregiver.

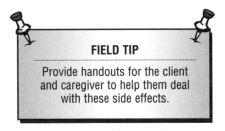

FIELD TIP

Provide handouts for the client and caregiver to help them deal with these side effects.

RIGHT TO SUPPORT OF FAMILY CAREGIVER

Even when highly motivated, the family caregiver experiences a great deal of stress. Friends and family members may be focusing so much on the client that they do not always recognize that the caregiver also needs support. The home health professional is responsible to assess not only how the care is being provided by the caregiver but also how well she/he is coping with the stress.

Sleep deprivation is a common problem encountered by the caregiver. If the client requires frequent attention, there may be constant sleep interruptions. It is helpful if there is more than one caregiver so they can take turns getting up to assist the client at night.

Caregivers report that they experience stress caused by the fear of causing harm, i.e., not knowing what to do to provide comfort or what to do at the time of death. They report that they do not know what questions to ask. We need to anticipate some of these issues and discuss them with the client and family members. Providing written information that will be available to the caregiver when needed is helpful.

Encourage caregivers to call the office when they have questions that cannot wait or when they need assistance. Assure them that someone will be available 24 hours a day. If the caregiver is having problems sharing concerns and stresses with other family members, you may be able to assist him/her by providing support while she/he talks with the family. There may be some respite assistance that can be provided. Observe the caregiver while providing care to evaluate the care and how well the caregiver is coping. Providing encouragement for the caregiver will ensure appropriate care for the client.

RIGHT TO A BROAD RANGE OF COVERED SERVICES

Originally the term hospice was used to identify a way station for travelers. Now the term defines an interdisciplinary program for terminally ill clients and their families. Hospice provides another alternative for care of the terminally ill client at home. The home health professional needs to determine if and when it is appropriate for the client to be referred to the hospice program. The implication is that the practitioner must be knowledgeable about the criteria for hospice care and share that information with the client and family caregiver.

The basic criteria for a hospice referral are a client diagnosed with a terminal illness and with a life expectancy of approximately six months. The client, the family, and physician all agree to participate in the program and no longer seek a curative treatment. There needs to be a primary care person available or some other alternative for physical care.

The client can elect to enroll in the hospice benefit program and may also choose to disenroll at any time. When enrolled, only hospice can be reimbursed for services related to the terminal illness. If treatment is required for an unrelated condition (e.g., fractured hip), a home health agency can receive reimbursement for those services.

If the client has been receiving care from the home health agency for some time, she/he may not wish to switch to hospice. The client and family must be fully informed of the services available to them through hospice so they can make an informed decision. They may need reassurance that they will not be disloyal to the home care agency if they choose to use hospice services.

Hospice services generally include skilled nursing, pain control, equipment and supplies, respite care, personal care, counseling, spiritual support, education and consultation services, volunteer services, bereavement care, information and resource materials. The hospice agency also provides 24-hour availability for emergency assistance.

Hospice agencies usually provide some of the specialized services, such as bereavement care, even if the client remains with the home health agency. It is important that you become knowledgeable about the hospice services in your geographic area and keep the client informed about those services.

RIGHT TO DIE IN PEACE AND DIGNITY

In addition to preparing the client and family for the moment of death, the nursing assistant, if helping in the client's care, needs to be prepared. She/he needs to know the aide's role when a client dies. First of all, the aide needs to know if the client has advanced directives and what are the client's wishes.

It helps if the client, family caregiver, and nursing assistant are informed about the signs of approaching death. They need to know that the last sense to leave the dying client is hearing. Encourage all caregivers to continue to talk to the client, even if she/he does not seem to respond. Family members can help the client by saying a favorite prayer so the client can hear it. Allow private moments for family members and any clergy, if desired, to spend with the client.

Other common physical changes as the client approaches death include:

  Slowed circulation, rapid, weak pulse, cold extremities
  Slowed respirations, noisy breathing
  Bladder and bowel incontinence
  Lost appetite and thirst.

RIGHT TO RESPECT OF BODY AFTER DEATH

If there is no physician's order or client consent for a do not resuscitate order, all resuscitative efforts that can be reasonably carried out must be done, and emergency assistance needs to be requested. After all appropriate emergency and life-saving measures have been followed in accordance with any advance directives, the CNA needs to phone the office, then remain with the client's body until the agency nurse arrives. It is hoped that there has been sufficient time for the family, with the help of the home care staff, to plan for all the needs that must be attended to based on the client's wishes.

State law dictates whether the registered nurse is able to pronounce the client dead or not. If the nurse does not have that authority, she/he will need to phone the physician to provide the assessment of life signs in order to obtain a pronouncement of death from the physician.

When the client is pronounced dead, the nursing assistant needs to prepare the body for the mortuary. The client's medication and any jewelry that may be on the client are turned over to the responsible family member. These actions need to be recorded in the visit note. A case communication form must be prepared to notify other agency staff members who were involved in the client's care of the client's death to prevent unnecessary phone calls or visits to the home during the bereavement period.

The home care professional can provide support to the family by assisting them with contacting the physician, funeral director, coroner, and next of kin, as appropriate. You can also provide assistance with spiritual concerns. Frequently, there has been sufficient time to help the client and family make funeral arrangements ahead of time, which helps to lessen the stress at the time of death. If the death has been anticipated, the agency could notify the coroner to expect their call. This lessens the coroner's inquiry at the actual time of death.

Assist the nursing assistant in the preparation of the body. Complete the necessary documentation including the pronouncement of death or the absence of vital signs, date, and time of death. A discharge summary and the appropriate OASIS documentation must be completed. Medicare will reimburse for a skilled nursing visit for pronouncement of death or assessment of life signs, depending on the state law, as long as it is not the only skilled nursing visit provided to the beneficiary.

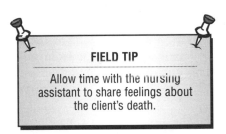

FIELD TIP

Allow time with the nursing assistant to share feelings about the client's death.

References

Agency for Health Care Policy and Research: Management of Cancer Pain: Adults, Pub # 94-0593. Washington D.C., U.S. Department of Health and Human Services, 1994.

Birchenall, J. and Streight, E.: Home Care Aide, pp. 425–430. St. Louis, Mosby-Year Book, 1997.

Brady, E. M.: Stories at the Hour of Our Death. Home Healthcare Nurse, 1999; 17(3):176–180.

Conley, V. M. and Burman, M. E.: Informational Needs of Caregivers of Terminal Patients in a Rural State. Home Healthcare Nurse, 1997; 15(11):808–817.

Davidhizar, R. and Dunn, C.: Malnutrition in the Elderly. Home Healthcare Nurse, 1996; 14(12):948–954.

Hospice of Yuma (Brochure). Yuma, Hospice of Yuma, 1997.

Johnson, D. L.: Pharmacologic Pain Management for Cancer Patients at Home. Home Healthcare Nurse, 1998; 16(3):166–173.

Kubler-Ross, E.: Death The Final Stage of Growth. Englewood Cliffs, NJ, Prentice-Hall, 1975.

Kubler-Ross, E.: On Death and Dying. New York, Macmillan Co., 1969.

Medicare Bulletin #419, by bcc (Blue Cross Calif) Fiscal Intermediary, Oxnard, CA, December 14, 1998, p. 11.

National Institutes of Health: Chemotherapy and You, 3rd edition, #92–1136. Washington, D.C., U.S. Department of Health and Human Services, 1991.

Olsten Health Services: Training and Development, OHM/Introduction to Medicare SSG, 1/97, pp. 1–6. Melville, NY, Olsten Health Services, 1997.

Olsten Health Services: Transitional Nurses Orientation Learner Guide, pp. 9-1 to 9-3. Melville, NY, Olsten Health Services, 1997.

Robert Wood Johnson Foundation: Strengthening Nursing Education to Improve Pain Management and End of Life Care. Duarte, CA, City of Hope National Medical Center, 1999.

Schall, M. B. and Faria, S. H.: Intervention Strategies to Alleviate Family Stressors. Home Care Provider, 1997; 2(6):315–318.

Safety Issues

Home health staff have safety issues, both personal and client related, that other health personnel do not even consider. This chapter explores various precautions that the nurse and therapist can use to protect themselves and their clients. The discussion is divided into three sections: Preparing for the Visit, Travel to and from Visits, and Safety During the Visit.

PREPARING FOR THE VISIT

When preparing for the visit, make sure the agency has your schedule for the day, and keep the agency informed if you make any changes in that schedule. If the agency knows where you are throughout the day, you can be reached in case a client, doctor, or your family needs to contact you. It also helps the agency to keep track of you in case you run into difficulties.

Most agencies will keep detailed directions to the clients homes on file. Make sure that you obtain the directions before you leave for the visit. A street map of the community in which you work is always a good idea to help find your way around. Call the client to make arrangements for the visit. This is also a good time to verify the directions to the home. If the client's residence is difficult to find or it is dark, it helps to ask the client or family to turn on an outside light. Frequently, they can give you some details to look for to make it easier to spot the home, such as a red car parked in front or a motor home parked on the side of the house.

It is a good idea to make sure you always carry a flash-light in case you are making a visit at night or before sun-rise. It is best to make your visits during daytime hours, but you don't always have that option. If you do have to make a visit at night and you are not sure about the neighborhood, ask for a family member to watch for your arrival. If the family has a menacing pet, ask them to make sure that the pet is tied up or closed up in a room.

Make sure that you have sufficient gas in your gas tank at all times. You never know when you may get lost and do not want to have to worry about running out of gas. Depending on the type of community in which you work, you may not have gas stations close by or you may be in a part of the community where you don't feel com-fortable stopping for gas. You will also want to keep your vehicle in good working order. Keep up with routine maintenance such as oil changes and checking tires for safety. Table 13–1 lists basic precautions to remember when preparing for a visit.

FIELD TIP

Always carry a street map and flashlight with extra batteries with you.

TRAVEL TO AND FROM THE VISIT

When traveling to and from the visit, keep in mind that you are a representative of your agency so drive safely and courteously. Do not carry a lot of money that could tempt someone, but make sure that you carry change so you can always phone the office if you get lost or have

Table 13-1	PREPARING FOR THE VISIT
	Keep agency informed about your schedule
	Get detailed directions to the client's home
	Carry a street map
	Verify appointment with client
	Carry a flashlight
	Have sufficient gas
	Keep vehicle in good working order

car problems. If you feel the need to carry a purse, lock it in the trunk of your car or put it somewhere so it is not visible. The same principles apply to your home health bag. Unfortunately, there are dishonest people in this world that think if you are a home health professional, you could be carrying drugs or drug paraphernalia in your bag.

Driving Precautions

Drive carefully and wear your seat belt when making visits. If you have five or six visits scheduled for the day and you are delayed at one of the earlier visits and want to get back on schedule, you may be tempted to rush more than is safe. You are better off not locking yourself into such a tight schedule that you are tempted to speed if you get off schedule. When scheduling your visits with clients, it is best to specify a range of time that you plan to arrive rather than commit to a particular time, such as between 10:30 AM and 11 AM rather than saying 11 AM.

Use your flashlight at night to read street signs or house numbers, so you do not need to get out of your car. Try to take well-traveled streets as much as possible. If you have car problems, pull over to the shoulder of the road, stay in the car, keep the car locked, and turn on your hazard lights. Towing insurance comes in handy for times like this. Some agencies provide cellular phones to their full-time professional employees. If not, it may still be worth the money for you to purchase you own cell phone. Wait until a police or security officer or someone you know arrives before you get out of the car, especially at night.

If you have a cell phone, remember that the use of the phone while driving seems to increase the risk of auto accidents. Drivers may become distracted when talking on the phone. Always pull over to the side of the road when you do need to use the phone.

Home health personnel need to be prepared to handle driving emergencies. Braking too sharply on a slippery roadway can put your vehicle into a skid. If the car does begin to skid, do not press the brake any further, and turn the wheel in the direction of the skid. As the car straightens out, turn the wheel back the other way, so it doesn't skid in the opposite direction. If your brakes fail, pump them rapidly. If this does not work, slowly apply the parking brake. Hold on to the brake release so you can ease off the brake in case the rear wheels lock. Shift to low gear and ease to a stop. If you have anti-lock brakes, do not pump them; just apply steady pressure. If you have a tire blow out, hold the steering wheel tightly to keep the vehicle going straight. Ease off the gas pedal; do not apply the brakes. Bring the vehicle to a gradual stop on the side of the road. A small fire extinquisher is handy to carry in case of a fire.

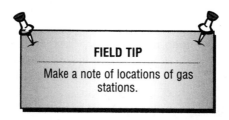

FIELD TIP

Make a note of locations of gas stations.

When you arrive at the client's residence, try to park close to the house. You want to limit the distance that you have to walk. Try to park in a well-lit area. Avoid parking on the client's property. This habit will help you avoid having an accident and causing property and car damage. There are times when you do not have the option of parking off the client's property. In that case be extra cautious.

When walking to and from the home, carry your keys in your hand. Then you do not have to fumble around looking for them when you want to enter your car. Try to stay on main thoroughfares. Make a lot of noise if you are ever accosted. Scream "Fire," "911," or "Help." If you see someone by your car, return to the client's home so you can phone for help.

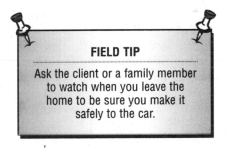

FIELD TIP

Ask the client or a family member to watch when you leave the home to be sure you make it safely to the car.

Always lock the car doors and keep the windows up. Do not leave anything of value in view. Do not wear expensive-looking jewelry. Keep your purse, wallet, and client folders locked in the car trunk, or if you do not have a trunk, put them out of sight such as under the car seat. Be sure that you carry in the needed supplies for the visit. When returning to your car, check the inside of your vehicle *before* entering it. In like fashion, be alert to the surrounding environment before you exit the car.

Intuition

Pay attention to your intuition and be aware of your surroundings. If the surroundings look suspicious or unsafe do not get out of the car. Avoid walking through a crowd of individuals. You might be mistaken, but it is not worth taking the risk. For example, you may drive up to the client's residence and observe a group of young men congregated in front of the home; if you have an uneasy feeling, you are safest by continuing to drive by. You can stop at a pay phone or use a cell phone to call either the office or the client. It may turn out that the young men are friends of the client's son or grandson. A simple phone call may be all that is needed to have the young men move on.

Aggressive Animals

Probably a greater hazard to home health personnel are animals, especially dogs. Dog bites tend to be a common employee injury for home health agencies. If you approach a home and discover a dog behaving protectively of the property, do not try to enter. Try calling to get the attention of the client or a family member to confine the dog. If you can't get anyone's attention, go to a pay phone or use your cell phone to call the family to lock up the animal. Once the agency is aware of a hazardous situation concerning an animal, the client and family must be instructed to always secure the animal whenever a member of the field staff is scheduled for an appointment. It is wise to remind the client of that agreement when you call to verify your appointment, at least until you are sure she/he will remember to secure the pet.

It is crucial that you communicate to the agency staff the possible danger of a protective animal. It is helpful to write a notation about the pet on the same form as the directions to the residence. Make a notation on the nursing assistants' care plans and also the forms made out for those who are covering on your days off to call their attention to the possible hazard.

During hot weather, make sure that you always have plenty of water with you. In winter weather, carry a snow shovel, ice scraper, and sand. Use extra caution driving during rainy and icy conditions. A set of jumper cables is useful no matter what the climate. If you make visits in remote areas, a sleeping bag, candles, and survival kit may come in handy. If you work in remote areas it is a good idea to carry a cell phone. Table 13–2 lists tips for traveling to and from a visit.

SAFETY DURING THE VISIT

Always knock before entering the home. It is better not to enter until the client or a family member acknowledges you. Identify yourself so they know who is there.

Volatile Situations

Be cautious about family situations which could escalate into dangerous situations. For example, if your client

Table 13–2	TRAVELING TO AND FROM VISITS

Do not carry a purse
Keep home health bag out of sight when left in car
Use defensive driving
Take precautions if your car breaks down
Park close to client's home
Park in well-lit areas
Always lock your car
Pay attention to your intuitive feelings
Be observant
Look in car before entering

and another family member begin to argue and the argument continues or becomes more intense, tell them that you do not feel comfortable and will have to leave if the argument continues. Frequently, saying this is all that is needed to defuse the situation. If the argument continues do not hesitate to leave. If you are concerned about the safety of the client, you can always call 911 after you leave the home. You will not be able to protect the client if you become injured. There have been instances when home health staff members have been injured in similar situations; in at least one instance, a staff member was shot because an argument got out of hand. Fortunately, the staff member who was shot was not killed.

Be aware of fire arms and other weapons that may be lying around the home. Occupational Safety and Health Administration (OSHA) now requires that agencies have a workplace violence prevention program. That policy needs to include a policy regarding fire arms, aggressive pets, and lethal substances such as acids. The agency policy is only as good as the willingness of the client to provide a safe environment and the field staffs' ability to assess for potential risks. There was one client who used to keep a hand gun by his bedside as a means of intimidating the caregivers. He refused to put the gun away so the agency informed him that they could no longer provide services.

When you visit a patient who seems to have the potential to be volatile, consider devising a plan in the event she/he should lose control. If you need guidance in such a situation, seek help from your supervisor. The social worker can also provide guidance in these situations. If the situation does escalate, be prepared to leave the home in a way that does not increase the danger.

Abuse or Neglect

Be alert for signs of abuse of the client. Abuse could be sexual, verbal, physical, or all of them. If you notice unexplained bruises, burns, scratches, broken bones, or suspicious scars or witness verbal abuse, you must take them seriously. The client may make statements that imply abuse or display fear of another person. If you suspect abuse, you are obligated to report your suspicions. Your supervisor can help you assess the situation.

If there is reason to believe that there is abuse, neglect, or exploitation of incapacitated or vulnerable adults or children occurring, the agency has a duty to report these concerns to the proper authorities. Some caregivers become concerned that they may be wrong about their suspicions of abuse, but they must still report their observations. It is the responsibility of the authorities to investigate whether or not there actually is abuse. There have been instances in which health care personnel have ignored signs of abuse, and a severe injury and even death have resulted. Health personnel are held more accountable for protecting their clients from abuse.

Health personnel are not obligated to allow abuse directed toward themselves. Verbal abuse is probably the most common type of abuse experienced by health care workers. There was a situation where a family member was verbally abusing several home health aides, but no one reported it because they each thought they must be doing something to invite the abuse. The agency was not able to handle the problem until the aides were willing to document the incidents. Each was surprised to learn that she/he was not the only one who was being abused. Table 13–3 lists precautions to be taken during the visit.

Table 13-3	SAFETY DURING THE VISITS
	Always knock before entering the residence
	Be cautious in unstable family situations
	Be alert for client abuse
	Protect your back
	Assess the home for unsafe features
	Be prepared for emergencies

Back Safety

OSHA has discontinued the requirement that a worker wear a back belt when lifting heavy objects or patients because they discovered that the use of a back belt could cause just as many problems as could be caused without the belt. If a caregiver wears the belt secured all of the time, even when not lifting, the back muscles eventually become weakened, which leads to a greater potential for back injury. Don't forget the greatest protection against back injury is the use of good body mechanics. As in health care facilities, a large number of employee injuries in home health are in the form of back injuries. Table 13–4 provides guidelines to protect your back.

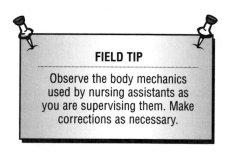

FIELD TIP

Observe the body mechanics used by nursing assistants as you are supervising them. Make corrections as necessary.

| Table 13–4 | GUIDELINES TO PROTECT YOUR BACK |

Push, pull, or roll a heavy object rather than lifting
Hold heavy objects close to you
Use longer and stronger muscles of legs rather than those of back
Use wide base of support
Keep back straight and bend knees
Point feet in direction you want to move
Do not twist upper part of your body
Clearly explain procedure to client
If client or object is too heavy, get help

Home Assessment

During the initial and subsequent visits, the client's home must be assessed to detect any unsafe features. Table 13–5 provides a list of major features to be evaluated during a home assessment.

You need to instruct the client and family about the importance of the features listed in Table 13–5. There was a client who was very unsteady on his feet. There was no stable fixture in the bathroom to provide support for him,

| Table 13–5 | MAJOR FOCI OF HOME ASSESSMENT |

Are there smoke alarms that work?
Do client and family have a plan for evacuation in case of fire?
Where are the exits located?
Are there scatter rugs that can cause falls?
Is there good lighting in the home?
Does the bathroom have grab bars, non-skid shower or tub surfaces, and shower or tub bench?
Is the home free of clutter?
Are medicines clearly labeled?
Are electrical cords in good working order?
Are electrical outlets free from overloading?

and he refused to have grab bars installed in the shower. He wanted to progress from a sponge bath to a shower, and that goal was used to motivate him to have the bars installed. Initially he was not happy, but he did get the grab bars installed and achieved his goal to shower.

Evacuation Plan

You want to help the family develop an evacuation plan in case of fire, and you always need a plan for yourself. If you anticipate various emergencies and mentally plan what you would do in case one arises, you will find that you are able to act appropriately in the given situation.

Always be alert to fire dangers. Locate the potential exits in the client's home and determine how you would get the client and yourself out safely. Some families try to save electricity when it is cold by turning on the stove's gas burners and oven, which puts them at risk for a fire. Teaching is required in a situation like this, but there may also be a need for a social work evaluation to assist the family so they don't have to worry about their heating bills. Make sure that the smoke detectors have working batteries in them. Some families forget to replace batteries and have a false sense of security that they will be warned in case of a fire.

Some other home features that can assist the client avoid injuries are clear pathways, a handy light at the bedside, and a phone near the bed. A soap on a rope in the shower or tub and a raised toilet seat are helpful. A night light in the bathroom is handy. If the family insists on having small rugs, non-skid backing will help prevent falls. Household cleaners and insecticides should remain in their original containers and should be kept out of reach of children. Remind clients and caregivers not to mix

cleaning solutions. The mixture could cause a poison-
ous gas.

Disasters

Each agency has its own plan in case of a disaster. The
nurse or therapist who admits a client is responsible for
rating the client in terms of their priority need for assistance if a disaster should occur.

Following is a example how clients can be prioritized.
Clients dependent on electricity, such as those receiving
oxygen or who are on a ventilator have top priority.
Those who require daily medication such as insulin-
dependent diabetics are rated second. Clients receiving
intravenous therapy or dressing changes are ranked
third. Those who are bedbound receive a fourth priority
rating. The fifth priority is for clients who are wheelchair-bound. The sixth priority is for someone who is
frail, fragile, or lives alone. All other clients are catego-
rized under the seventh priority, other.

If the client fits into more than one category, rank
him/her in the highest priority. An example would be a
client who is receiving oxygen and is wheelchair-bound.
She/he should be ranked as priority one.

Client classifications also indicate if they have a visual,
auditory, speech, or total sensory deficit. Priority status
is indicated for clients who fit into more than one these
classifications. For example, a client who is blind, lives
alone, and requires daily insulin has ranking of V for visual, 2 priority for insulin need, and PS for priority
status.

The administrative nurse on call needs to carry a list of all
the agency's clients and their ratings with him/her at all
times. If there is some type of disaster, such as flooding or
a power outage, the nurse will initiate the disaster plan.

The top priority clients will be called to see if they have electricity or need any assistance. The oxygen-dependent clients will be checked to be sure they have back-up oxygen systems. These back-up systems should always be in place. The administrative nurse will obtain assistance with phone calls so all of the clients can be contacted as the situation dictates. The field staff will be contacted as necessary to assist the clients.

Emergency Situations in the Home

Nurses in acute or extended care facilities always have other health care personnel around to help in emergencies. In the home, you must rely on your own professional judgment and agency policies.

Of course if the client has signed a Do Not Resuscitate (DNR) order or has a living will, you have to act accordingly. You would want to help the client and family anticipate problems and discuss what they can do if the situation should arise. For example, if the client is prone to have seizures, discuss with the client and family members what the seizure would look like and what they can do to protect the client. Encourage the family members to share how they would feel if the situation would materialize. Once they understand how to protect the client, they usually feel more comfortable about caring for him.

Just because the client has a DNR order does not mean that she/he should never receive emergency treatment. For example, a client who falls and injures a hip is still going to require treatment.

In case of an emergency with a client who does not have a DNR order, such as a serious fall or chest pain, call 911. If the client has a respiratory or cardiac arrest, of course you would follow the procedure for CPR, which includes calling 911.

The teaching plan for home health clients should include procedures to follow in case of emergencies. Any nurse who handles the evening and weekend phone calls from clients will frequently run into a situation when a client or family member calls to say that the client is having chest pain or some other emergency. It is best to instruct him/her to hang up and call 911. Then have him/her call back when assistance has been obtained. If you do not hear from him/her, call back to make sure she/he received help. You may be tempted to phone 911 yourself, but the family member can give better directions to the home. Emergency personnel can provide some instructions via phone that the family member can do while waiting for the ambulance. Also, if the client or family member panics and hangs up before giving detailed directions to the house, the 911 system can trace the call.

When you call 911, be the last one to hang up the phone. Sometimes you think that you have given the dispatcher sufficient information but she/he may have some more questions. Once there was an emergency call requesting paramedics for a client having chest pain. The caller gave the address for a mobile home park that had over 100 mobile home spaces but forgot to give the space number. The ambulance had to waste precious moments trying to find the correct place.

It is helpful if someone stays out in front of the home to flag down the ambulance. That someone should not be you. Your first responsibility is to the client. You must remain with the client until you can turn over the care to a paramedic. If you are performing CPR, expect to continue for awhile after the paramedics arrive because they will need to get set up before they can take over total care. Once the client is on the way to the hospital, do not forget to phone the office to inform the agency of what happened.

Table 13–6	PREPARATION FOR EMERGENCIES AND DISASTERS
	Know the agency's disaster plan
	Prioritize the client's disaster rating accurately
	Formulate a plan for emergencies
	Determine an evacuation plan in case of fire

All field staff are expected to carry a CPR mask device with them when making visits. You may think that you won't need to worry about CPR for a particular client because the client has a DNR order, but what if something happens to another family member? Table 13–6 lists measures to take in preparation for disasters and emergencies.

This chapter discussed some of the major safety situations encountered by home health personnel. There is no way all possible circumstances can be anticipated. By taking safety precautions and using common sense, home care staff should remain safe.

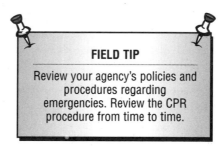

FIELD TIP

Review your agency's policies and procedures regarding emergencies. Review the CPR procedure from time to time.

References

AHCCCS Fraud Control Unit: Abuse, Neglect, and Exploitation of the Elderly, pp. 2–10. Phoenix, Office of Arizona Attorney General, 1996.

American Association of Retired Persons: 55 Alive Mature Driving, pp. 48–56. Washington, D.C., AARP, 1994.

Arizona Department of Motor Vehicles: Arizona Driver License Manual, pp. 46–48. Phoenix, Motor Vehicle Division, 1998.

Arizona Revised Statutes: 1995 Cumulative Pocket Part, 5A; 13–3620 to 46–455. St. Paul, MN, West Publishing, 1995.

Birchenall, J. and Streight, E.: Home Care Aide, pp. 168–169, St. Louis, Mosby-Year Book, 1997.

Dixon, B.T.: Help Patients Make Their Homes User-Friendly. Private Duty Homecare, 1998; Jan:13–14.

Hunter, E.: Violence Prevention in the Home Health Setting. Home Healthcare Nurse, 1997; 15(6):403–408.

Lacey, M.: Recognizing Patterns of Child Abuse in the Home. Home Care Provider, 1998; 3(6):319–322.

Morrison, B.: Home Health Care—Staying Safe in Dangerous Times. Nursing 1995; Oct:49–51.

Safety: Use 6 tips to teach staff "street smarts." Homecare Education Management, 1996; 1(1):5–11.

Olsten Health Services: Training and Development, Aide-level training Program, Module 1.97, Melville, N.Y., Olsten Health Services, 1997, pp. 1–2 to 1–5.

Prevent Weather-Related Accidents in the Winter. Homecare Education Management, 1996; 1(12):167–169.

Wagner, L.: Home Safety for Elders. Home Health Focus, 1997; 4(4):27.

Wilson, T. H.: OSHA Guide for Health Care Facilities, Sec 753. Washington, D.C., Occupational Safety and Health Administration, 1998.

Body Systems Review

HEENT*

Glasses
Contact lenses
Cataracts
Glaucoma
Impaired hearing
Dentures/partials

CARDIOVASCULAR

Apical pulse
Edema
Peripheral pulses
Neck vein disten-
tion
Calf tenderness
Varicose veins
Chest pain
Arrhythmia
Hypertension
Myocardial infarction
Deep venous throm-
bosis
Pacemaker
Vertigo/syncope
Congestive heart
failure
Orthostatic hypoten-
sion

ENDOCRINE/ METABOLIC

Diabetes
Thyroid problems
Blood test meter
Jaundice

GASTRO- INTESTINAL

Abdomen
description
tenderness
Blood sugar
Appetite/hydration
Nausea
Vomiting
Diarrhea/
constipation
Distention
Ascites
Dysphagia
Incontinent
Hemorrhoids
Laxative use
Bleeding
Hernia
Ostomy
Cancer
Gallbladder disease

Ulcers
Gastric tube

MUSCULO- SKELETAL

Range of motion
Swollen joints
Bone/muscle pain
Deformity
Stiffness
Arthritis
Osteoporosis
Neuropathy
Fractures
Paralysis
Atrophy
Gait/falls
Transfers
Immobility
Amputation
Prosthesis

NEUROLOGIC

Altered levels of con-
sciousness
Sensation
Tremors
Paralysis

Cognitive change
Weakness
Unsteady gait
Vertigo/syncope
Grips
Perla†
Headache
Seizures
Transient ischemia
   attacks
Cerebrovascular acci-
   dent
Parkinson's disease

RESPIRATORY

Breath sounds
Cough/sputum
Chronic obstructive
   pulmonary disease
Tuberculosis

Asthma
Dyspnea
Orthopnea
Nail bed color
Pain
Nebulizer
Tracheotomy
Oxygen therapy

SURGERIES

Record each one and
   dates

GENITOURINARY

Pain, frequency, ur-
   gency
Burning, inconti-
   nence
Nocturia

Hematuria
Bleeding/discharge
Renal failure
Infections
Kidney stones
Prostate problems
Sexually active
Pregnancy
Breast examination

INTEGUMENTARY

Turgor
Lacerations
Abrasions
Bruises
Rash
Ulcers
Color
General Condition

---

* Head, eyes, ears, nose, throat
† Pupils equal, round; reaction to light; accommodation

Home Health Certification and Plan of Care Form (HCFA-485)

B

Department of Health and Human Services
Health Care Financing Administration

EXHIBIT I

Form Approved
OMB No. 0938-0357

HOME HEALTH CERTIFICATION AND PLAN OF TREATMENT

1. Patient's HI Claim No.	2. SOC Date	3. Certification Period		4. Medical Record No.	5. Provider No.
		From:	To:		

6. Patient's Name and Address	7. Provider's Name and Address

8. Date of Birth:		9. Sex ☐ M ☐ F	10. Medications: Dose/Frequency/Route (N)ew (C)hanged
11. ICD-9-CM	Principal Diagnosis	Date	
12. ICD-9-CM	Surgical Procedure	Date	
13. ICD-9-CM	Other Pertinent Diagnoses	Date	

14. DME and Supplies	15. Safety Measures:
16. Nutritional Req.	17. Allergies:

18. A. Functional Limitations

1 ☐ Amputation	5 ☐ Paralysis	9 ☐ Legally Blind	
2 ☐ Bowel/Bladder (Incontinence)	6 ☐ Endurance	A ☐ Dyspnea with Minimal Exertion	
3 ☐ Contracture	7 ☐ Ambulation	B ☐ Other (Specify)	
4 ☐ Hearing	8 ☐ Speech		

18. B. Activities Permitted

1 ☐ Complete Bedrest	6 ☐ Partial Weight Bearing	A ☐ Wheelchair	
2 ☐ Bedrest BRP	7 ☐ Independent At Home	B ☐ Walker	
3 ☐ Up as Tolerated	8 ☐ Crutches	C ☐ No Restrictions	
4 ☐ Transfer Bed/Chair	9 ☐ Cane	D ☐ Other (Specify)	
5 ☐ Exercise Prescribed			

19. Mental Status:

1 ☐ Oriented	3 ☐ Forgetful	5 ☐ Disoriented	7 ☐ Agitated
2 ☐ Comatose	4 ☐ Depressed	6 ☐ Lethargic	8 ☐ Other

20. Prognosis

1 ☐ Poor	2 ☐ Guarded	3 ☐ Fair	4 ☐ Good	5 ☐ Excellent

21. Orders for Discipline and Treatments (Specify Amount/Frequency/Duration)

22. Goals/Rehabilitation Potential/Discharge Plans

23. Nurse's Signature and Date of Verbal SOC Where Applicable:	25. Date HHA Received Signed POT
24. Physician's Name and Address	26. I certify/recertify that this patient is confined to his/her home and needs intermittent skilled nursing care, physical therapy and/or speech therapy or continues to need occupational therapy. The patient is under my care, and I have authorized the services on this plan of care and will periodically review the plan.
27. Attending Physician's Signature and Date Signed	28. Anyone who misrepresents, falsifies, or conceals essential information required for payment of Federal funds may be subject to fine, imprisonment, or civil penalty under applicable Federal laws.

Form HCFA-485 (C-4) (02-94) PROVIDER

Bibliography

About Standard Precautions, pp. 1–15. Deerfield, MA, Channing L. Bete Co., 1997.

About Infection Control in the Home, pp. 1–15. Deerfield, MA, Channing L. Bete Co., 1995.

Agency for Health Care Policy and Research: Management of Cancer Pain: Adults, Pub # 94-0593. Washington D.C., U.S. Department of Health and Human Services, 1994.

AHCCCS Fraud Control Unit: Abuse, Neglect, and Exploitation of the Elderly, pp. 2–10. Phoenix, Office of Arizona Attorney General, 1996.

A Homecare Therapist Guide to Medicare Service Delivery. The Beacon Homecare FOCUS Series. Medicare Reimbursement for Therapy Services, pp. 1–9, Mequon, WI, Beacon Health, 1996.

American Association of Retired Persons: 55 Alive Mature Driving, pp. 48–56. Washington, D.C., AARP, 1994.

Arizona Association for Home Care: OASIS Alert, June 18. Phoenix, AAHC, 1999.

Arizona Association for Home Care: Update: 15-Minute Increment Reporting. March 12. Phoenix, Arizona Association for Home Care, 1999.

Arizona Certified Agency Policy Manuel: COP Interpretive Guidelines for Home Health Agencies, pp. B–13 to B–20. Phoenix, Department of Health Services, 1997.

Arizona Department of Motor Vehicles: Arizona Driver License Manual, pp. 46–48. Phoenix, Motor Vehicle Division, 1998.

Arizona Revised Statutes: 1995 Cumulative Pocket Part, 5A; 13–3620 to 46–455. St. Paul, MN, West Publishing, 1995.

Avoiding Fraud & Abuse Charges: The Beacon Homecare FOCUS Series, Medicare Reimbursement for Therapy Services, pp. 15–16. Mequon, WI, Beacon Health, 1996.

Benner, M.: Congress Approves Minimal Changes to Medicare Home Health Benefit. Home Care Provider 1998; 3 (6): 312–313.

Benner, M.: The Medicare Interim Payment System's Impact on Home Health Services. Home Care Provider 1998; 3(3): 169–170.

Birchenall, J. and Streight, E.: Home Care Aide, pp. 168–169. St. Louis, Mosby-Year Book, 1997.

Blanchard, L., Gill, G., and Williams, E.: Guidelines and Documentation Requirements for Social Workers in Home Health Care, Chapters 3 & 8. Silver Spring, MD, National Association of Social Workers, 1991.

Brady, E. M.: Stories at the Hour of Our Death. Home Healthcare Nurse 1999; 17(3):176–180.

Calfee, B.: Labor Laws Working to Protect You. Nursing 96; 26(2):34–39.

Can You Pass Home Healthcare Nurse's OASIS Quiz? Home Healthcare Nurse 1999; 17(1):60–61.

Ceslowitz, S. B. and Loreti, S. T.: Easing the Transition from Hospital Nursing to Home Care: A Research Study. Home Healthcare Nurse, 1991; 9(4):32–35.

Conley, V. M. and Burman, M. E.: Informational Needs of Caregivers of Terminal Patients in a Rural State. Home Healthcare Nurse, 1997; 15(11):808–817.

Crisler, K. S.: Oasis: What it is and How to Implement and Integrate it in a Home Care Agency, pp. 1–11. Denver, Center for Health Services and Policy Research, 1998.

Czarnik, B.: Medicare Coverage Issues. Home Healthcare Nurse 1997; 15(7):512–514.

Danks, S. A.: Building Relationships with Medicare Managed-Care Case Managers. Home Healthcare Nurse 1999; 17(1):53–56.

Davidbizar, R. and Dunn, C.: Malnutrition in the Elderly. Home Healthcare Nurse, 1996; 14(12):948–954.

Determining Homebound Status. The Beacon Homecare FOCUS Series, pp. 1–14. Mequon, WI, Beacon Health, 1996.

Dixon, B. T.: Help patients make their homes user-friendly. Private Duty Homecare 1998; Jan:13–14.

Dreyer, C. J.: Home Health Aide Supervision: Care Plans and Supervisory Visits. Home Health FOCUS 1998; 5(6):45.

Epley, D. and Faria, S. H.: Assessment of Infections in Home Care Patients. Home Care Provider 1999; 4(1):13–16.

Fraud and Abuse in the Home Health Services Field. AHA Legal Alert, pp. 1–3. Washington, D.C., American Hospital Association, 1997.

Garity, J.: Gender Differences in Learning Style of Alzheimer Family Caregivers. Home Healthcare Nurse 1999; 17(1): 37–43.

Glasser, C. R.: Managing Functional Limitations. Home Health FOCUS, 1998; 4(12):89.

Gorski, L. A.: Case Management: Collaboration is Essential. Home Health FOCUS 1998; 5(5):38.

1998 Grolier Multimedia Encyclopedia. U.S. Department of Health and Human Services, Danbury, CT, Grolier Interactive Inc., 1998.

1998 Grolier Multimedia Encyclopedia. Social and Welfare Services. Danbury, CT, Grolier Interactive Inc., 1998.

Hanneken, K.: OASIS Update. AAHC Arizona Homefront 1998; 15(11):1.

Harris, M. D.: Medicare and the Nurse. Home Healthcare Nurse 1998; 16(11):732–736.

Harris, M.: The Physician as a Member of the Home Healthcare Team. Home Healthcare Nurse 1998; 16(11):732–735.

Hartley, W. and Vincent, W.: American Civics, 4th edition, pp. 43–45, pp. 122–129. Orlando, Harcourt Brace Jovanovich, 1983.

Health Care Financing Administration: BBA Implementation Tracking Report. Available at: http://www.hcfa.gov

Health Care Financing Administration: Home Health Agency Manual (HIM-11), Coverage of Services, Sec 200-220, pp. 11–24. Washington, D.C., Department of Health and Human Services, 1987.

Health Care Financing Administration: Home Health Agency Manual (HIM-11) General Information about the Program, Sec 100, pp. 6–8. Washington, D.C., Department of Health and Human Services, 1992.

Health Care Financing Administration: Home Health Agency Manual (HIM-11) Coverage of Services, Sec 200-230, pp. 11–24. Washington, D.C., Department of Health and Human Services, 1996.

Health Care Financing Administration: Home Health Agency Manual (HIM-11) Coverage of Services, Sec 234, pp. 11–24. Washington, D.C., Department of Health and Human Services, 1998.

Health Care Financing Administration: OASIS Implementation Manual, Attachment A, General OASIS Instructions, pp. 8.11–8.12. Washington, D.C., Department of Health and Human Services, 1998.

Health Care Financing Administration: OASIS Implementation Manual, Attachment, B, pp. 8.62–8.75. Washington D.C., Department of Health and Human Services, 1998.

Hefty, L.V., Kenyon, V., Martaus, T., et al.: A Model Skills List for Orienting Nurses to Community Health Agencies. Public Health Nursing 1992; 9(4):228–233.

Hilliard, L. S.: Manager's Corner: Innovative or Disintegrate. Home Care Nurse News 1998; 5(6):1–2, 8.

Hogue, E.: Avoiding Liability for Abandonment in an Environment of Reduced Medicare Utilization. Arizona Homefront 1998; 15(3):5–7.

Hogue, E.: Avoiding Liability for Termination of Services/Abandonment (Handout). Burtonsville, MD, 1998.

Hogue, E. E.: Communications with Physicians (Handout). Burtonsville, MD, 1998.

Hogue, E.: HCFA Addresses Issues Related to Termination of Services. Arizona Homefront 1998; 15(9):6–7.

Hogue, E.: How to Deal with Today's Challenges of Managing Patient Mix. Arizona Homefront 1999; 16(2):6.

Hogue, E.: The Behavioral Offset of the Interim Payment System: What HCFA Expects Home Care Providers to do. Arizona Homefront 1998; 15(6):10–11.

Home Care 101: The Patient Controls the Home. Homecare Education Management 1996; 1(1):1–3.

Home Health Compliance Risk Areas as Identified by the OIG: Home Care Compliance Alert 1998; 2(9):108.

Hospice of Yuma (Brochure). Yuma, Hospice of Yuma, 1997.

Hospital and Payor ICD-9-CM, Vol 1, 2, 3. Salt Lake City, Medicode Inc., 1998.

Hunter, E.: Violence prevention in the Home Health Setting. Home Healthcare Nurse 1997; 15(6):403–408.

Johnson, D. L.: Pharmacologic Pain Management for Cancer Patients at Home. Home Healthcare Nurse 1998; 16(3): 166–173.

Johnson, J. (Ed.): Medicare Fraud and Abuse: Understanding the Law. Introduction. Washington, D.C., National Health Lawyers Association, 1986.

Keating, S. B.: Infection Control in the Home Setting. Home Care Provider 1999; 4(1):4.

Kenyon, V., Smith, E., Hefty, L. V., et al.: Clinical Competencies for Community Health Nursing. Public Health Nursing 1990; 7(1):33–39.

Knowles, M.: The Modern Practice of Adult Education. New York, Association Press, 1970.

Kubler-Ross, E.: Death The Final Stage of Growth. Englewood Cliffs, NJ, Prentice-Hall, 1975.

Kubler-Ross, E.: On Death and Dying. New York, Macmillan Co., 1969.

Lacey, M.: Recognizing Patterns of Child Abuse in the Home. Home Care Provider 1998; 3(6):319–322.

Law Watch: A Legal Newsletter. Chicago, Foley Lardner Weissburg & Aronson, 1998.

Long, C. O., Ismeurt, R. L., and White, P. A.: Preventing Drug Interactions in the Home: A Five-Step Approach for Client Teaching. Home Healthcare Nurse 1999; 17(2):106–112.

Management and Evaluation of a Care Plan: The Beacon Homecare FOCUS Series, pp. 1–16. Mequon, WI, Beacon Health, 1996.

Martin, J. P.: Home Care Orientation Manual. California Association for Health Services at Home. Sacramento, 1995.

Mason, J. E. and Hansen, J. F.: Teaching and Learning: An Overview, pp. 1–10. Patient Teaching Loose-leaf Library. Springhouse, PA, Springhouse Corp., 1991.

Medicare Bulletin #413, by bbc (Blue Cross Calif) Fiscal Intermediary, Oxnard, CA, January 15, p. 8, 1998.

Medicare Bulletin #414, by bbc (Blue Cross Calif) Fiscal Intermediary, Oxnard, CA, March 25, p. 12, 1998.

Medicare Bulletin #415. by bcc (Blue Cross Calif) Fiscal Intermediary, Oxnard, CA, May 4, 1998.

Medicare Bulletin #416, by bcc (Blue Cross Calif) Fiscal Intermediary, Oxnard, CA, July 13, p. 13, 1998.

Medicare Bulletin #419, by bcc (Blue Cross Calif) Fiscal Intermediary, Oxnard, CA, December 14, p. 11, 1998.

Medicare Reimbursement of Therapy Services: The Beacon Homecare FOCUS Series, pp. 1–9. Mequon, WI, Beacon Health, 1996.

Milone-Nuzzo, P.: Beyond Venipuncture as the Qualifying Service for Medicare: Seeing the Forest for the Trees. Home Healthcare Nurse 1998; 16(3):177–178.

Morrison, B.: Home Health Care: Staying Safe in Dangerous Times. Nursing 1995; Oct:49–51.

Narayan, M. C.: Survey Highlights the Concerns of Home Healthcare Nurses. Home Healthcare Nurse 1999; 17(1):57.

National Association for Home Care: HIM-11 Coverage Guide for Field Staff. Washington, D.C., National Association for Home Care, 1998.

National Institutes of Health: Chemotherapy and You, 3rd edition, #92-1136. Washington, D.C., Department of Health and Human Services, 1991.

Neighbors, M. and Monahan, F. D.: A Practical Guide to Medical-Surgical Nursing in the Home, sections 1 & 6, pp. 48–55, 668–673. Philadelphia, W. B. Saunders Co, 1998.

Nelson, S.: The Importance of an Infection Control Program in Home Care. Arizona Homefront 1999; 16(2):5.

Nicoll, L. H.: Nurses' Guide to the Internet, 2nd edition. Philadelphia, Lippincott, 1998.

Nissenboim, S. and Vroman, C. The Positive Interactions: Programs of Activities for People with Alzheimer's Disease. Baltimore, Health Professions Press, 1998.

Olsten Health Services: Client Care Management for Hospital Alliance Home Health Agencies. Documentation Protocols, pp. 4-1 to 4-9, Supervision, pp. 10–6 to 10–8. Tampa, FL, Olsten Management Services, 1995.

Olsten Health Services: Continuing Nurses Education. pp. 12–5 to 12–15. Melville, NY, Olsten Health Services, 1996.

Olsten Health Services: Training and Development, Aide-level Training Program, Module 1, 1/97, pp. 1–2 to 1–5. Melville, NY, Olsten Health Services, 1997.

Olsten Health Services: Training and Development, OHM/Introduction to Medicare SSG, 1/97, pp. 1–3 to 1–17, 3–3 to 3–10, 4–3 to 4–6. Melville, NY, Olsten Health Services, 1997.

Olsten Health Services: Transitional Nurses Orientation Learner Guide, pp. 3–5 to 6–15, 7–1 to 7–14, 9–1 to 9–3, 10–2 to 10–8. Melville, NY, Olsten Health Services, 1997.

Pearson, M. and Wessman, J.: Gerogogy in Patient Education. Home Healthcare Nurse 1996; 14(8):631–636.

Perry, S. and Shipes, E.: Collecting Assessment Data, pp. 11–30. Patient Teaching Loose-leaf Library. Springhouse, PA, Springhouse Corp., 1991.

Peterson, E. and Solomon, D.: Maintaining Healthy Boundaries in Pressional Relationships: A Balancing Act. Home Care Provider 1998; 3(6):314–318.

Polzien, G., Kendall, B., and Hindelang, M.: The challenge of implementing OASIS. Home Healthcare Nurse, 1998; 16(12):806–812.

Popovich, M.: A Look Back at 10 Years of Home Care Accreditation at the Joint Commission. Home Care Provider 1998; 3(6):326–328.

Popovich, M. L.: The Joint Commission's Home Care Standards for Infection Control. Home Care Provider 1999; 4(1): 40–41.

Popovich, M.: Why Become Accredited? Benefits and Values of Joint Commission Accreditation. Home Care Provider 1998; 3(3):173–175.

Prevent Weather-Related Accidents in the Winter: Homecare Education Management 1996; 1(12):167–169.

Rimmer, L. M.: What Every Home Healthcare Nurse Should Know About Complementary Therapy. Home Healthcare Nurse 1998; 16(11):760–764.

Robert Wood Johnson Foundation: Strengthening Nursing Education to Improve Pain Management and End of Life Care. Duarte, CA, City of Hope National Medical Center, 1999.

Rowe, P. and Tackenberg, J. N.: Implementing the Teaching Plan, pp. 43–48. Patient Teaching Loose-leaf Library. Springhouse, PA, Springhouse Corp., 1991.

Rowe, P. and Wells, E. A.: Planning for Teaching, pp. 31–42. Patient Teaching Loose-leaf Library. Springhouse, PA, Springhouse Corp., 1991.

Safety: Use 6 Tips to Teach Staff "Street Smarts." Homecare Education Management 1996; 1(1):5–11.

Salminen, C.: Designating Your Compliance Officer. AAHC Arizona Homefront 1998; 15(11):1.

Salminen, C.: (Yet another) Corporate Compliance Update. AAHC Arizona Homefront 1998; 15(10):5.

Schall, M. B. and Faria, S. H.: Intervention Strategies to Alleviate Family Stressors. Home Care Provider 1997; 2(6): 315–318.

Schmid, M. M. and Liaschenko, J.: Ethical Issues in Infection Control in Home Care. Home Care Provider 1999; 4(1):8–9.

Schroeder, B.: Medicare Case Management. Home Health FOCUS 1998; 5(1):5.

Setting the Record Straight: An Industry Response to Fraud and Abuse. Homecare, pp. 19–20. Washington D.C., National Association for Home Care, 1998.

Sherry, D.: Time Management Strategies of the New Home Care Nurse. Home Healthcare Nurse 1996; 14(9):718–720.

Sitzman, K.: Tips for Using OASIS. Home Healthcare Nurse 1998; 16(8):561.

Snow, L., Hefty, L. V., Kenyon, V., et al.: Making the Fit: Orienting New Employees to Community Health Nursing Agencies. Public Health Nursing 1992; 9(1):58–64.

Sommer, B.: Protecting our Patients and Ourselves. Home Care Provider 1999; 4(1):30–33.

Sperling, R.: How OASIS Relates to the Medicare 485. Home Healthcare Nurse 1999; 17(2):82–85.

Sperling, R.: What's this OASIS, Anyway? Home Healthcare Nurse 1998; 16(6):373–374.

Stempel, J.: Pain Management in Terminal Illness. Home Health FOCUS 1997; 4(3):17–19.

Stewart, M.: New Law Eases Medicare Interim Payment System Burden on Home Health Care. The American Nurse 1998; Nov/Dec:10.

Stoker, J.: Congress's Report Card on Home Care Progress. Home Healthcare Nurse 1999; 17(3):158.

Stoker, J.: Defining Homebound Status. Home Healthcare Nurse 1999; 17(2):119.

Stoker, J.: Home Care Voices Heard. Home Healthcare Nurse 1999; 17(1):8.

Stoker, J.: OASIS as a Mandatory Medicare Requirement. Home Healthcare Nurse 1998; 16(9):595.

Stoker, J.: The Regulatory Changes of 1998. Home Healthcare Nurse 1998; 16(11):740.

Stonerock, C.: Home Health Aides: Home Care's "Endangered Species." Home Care Provider 1997; 2(1):15–17.

Thobaben, M.: Understanding the Internet and World Wide Web. Home Care Provider 1999; 4(4):10–12.

Thomas, M. N.: Understanding Medicare Reimbursement. Home Healthcare Nurse 1998; 16(12):840–843.

Top "Dos and Don'ts" of Private Duty Home Care: Eli's Home Health Line, 1999; March 29:10–11.

Touchard, B. M. and Berthelot, K.: Collaborative Home Practice: Nursing and Occupational Therapy Ensure Appropriate Medication Administration. Home Healthcare Nurse 1999; 17(1):45–51.

Transitioning to Home Care: Follow these 6 Tips to Orient Ex-hospital Nurses. Homecare Education Management 1996; 1(1):1–3.

Wagner, L.: Home Safety for Elders. Home Health Focus 1997; 4(4):27.

Weissenstein, E.: Home Health "Guidelines" include Mandates. Modern Healthcare 1998; Aug: 6.

Wellmark Fiscal Intermediary: Medicare Guide to Billing for HHAs, pp. 1–22. Des Moines, IA, Wellmark, Inc., 1997.

Western Arizona Council of Governments: Area Agency on Aging Services Information Pamphlet, pp. 6–9. Yuma, AZ, WACOG, 1997.

Wilkinson, J. M.: Nursing diagnosis and intervention pocket guide, 6th edition. Menlo Park, Addison-Wesley Co., 1995.

Wilson, T. H.: OSHA Guide for Health Care Facilities, Sec. 513, 523, 753, Appendix I. Washington, D.C., Occupational Safety and Health Administration, 1998.

Woods, G.: Telephone Scams and Older Consumers (brochure). Phoenix, Arizona Office of the Attorney General, 1995.

Yuan, J. R.: Using Standards and Guidelines in Your Daily Practice. Home Healthcare Nurse 1998; 16(11):753–759.

Index

Page numbers followed by t refer to illustrations.